Living Life as Parent-Partners

By Merle H. Weiner

Professor of Law
and
Author of *A Parent-Partner Status for American Family Law* (Cambridge University Press 2015)

© Merle H. Weiner, 2015

For the children of my parent-partnership, Eli and Henry.

Living Life as Parent-Partners

Introduction

Congratulations on purchasing these practical instructions for how to live your life as a "parent-partner."

A "parent-partner" is the term used to describe the relationship between two people who have a child in common. It is not a legal term — or even a term that would be recognized by most people in society — although it should be both.

Two people with a child in common become parent-partners automatically, regardless of whether they are in a romantic relationship, they are married, or they want to be parent-partners. The term "parent-partner" describes the social role that each parent acquires when he or she has or adopts a child. That role defines the parent's relationship with the other parent. The role lasts throughout a person's lifetime, just like the social role of "parent."

Although any two people with a child in common are parent-partners, the term is used throughout this book to suggest that the couple has a solid parent-partnership. "Living Life as Parent-Partners" means living life as good parent-partners, not as bad parent-partners. Imagine if you bought a book entitled, *Becoming a Parent*. The author would not describe how to be a neglectful or abusive parent, but rather would describe how to be the parent that the child needs and that society expects.

Unfortunately, society currently expects very little of parent-partners. Society should expect parent-partners to act as a supportive, cooperative team from the get-go and throughout their child's life. If such expectations existed, people would make better decisions about when and with whom to have a child. Society's expectations would also encourage parents to work hard to keep their relationships with the other parent vibrant, healthy, and strong. These results would allow parents be the sort of parenting team that children need!

The following recommendations are informed by the expectations that society *should* have for parent-partners, and that *you* should have for your own parent-partnership.

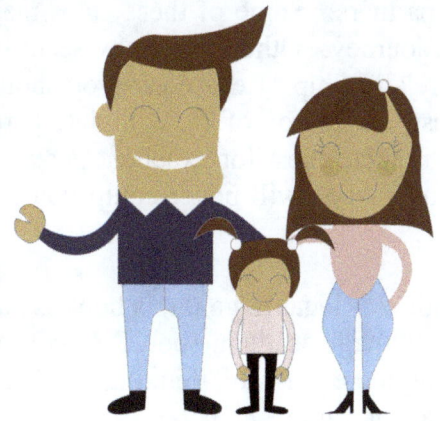

This book is a companion to a scholarly book entitled, *A Parent-Partner Status for American Family Law*, published by Cambridge University Press in 2015. That book focuses on law, theory, and social change. Frankly, that book is a bit eggheady.

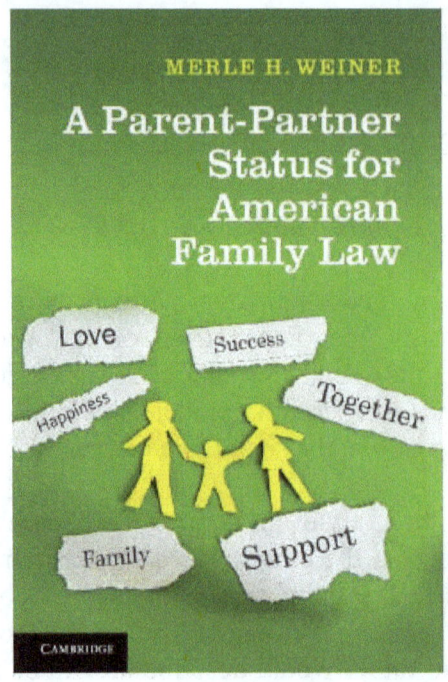

In contrast, this book is written to inform a general audience about the "parent-partner" concept. It is a "how-to" guide and is designed for people who want to follow the philosophy of the parent-partner status on a personal level, regardless of whether legal or social change ever occurs.

This book is filled with information about what living life as a good parent-partner requires. It tells you why living life as a good parent-partner is best for you and your child. It also gives you tips for living your life in a way that is consistent with the values underlying the parent-partner concept. This book concludes with some ideas for how you can help the parent-partner concept catch on so that all children might have the advantage of parents who act like parent-partners.

In the pages that follow, you will find a description of twenty steps that you and your partner can take to live life fully as parent-partners. Some of these steps may not apply to you if you are further along on the parenthood journey. Other steps may seem like they will never be needed because of the strength of your relationship. Regardless, you should still review all of the steps. Reading the entire book will best inform you of the complete parent-partner concept. Doing so will also help you guide others in their quest for excellent parent-partnerships. Additionally, if you like the idea, reading the entire book will better equip you to advocate for laws that could make this concept catch on faster.

Although this book has no footnotes or legal jargon, this book is based on extensive research and informed by the analysis in the 600-page academic book. Don't mistake this book's brevity and matter-of-fact tone with fluff or mere wishful thinking. What follows has substance, and hopefully you will find that it also has value.

Should I read this book?

After all, reading a book takes time away from other activities. If you already have a child, your free time may be extremely limited already, making this question even more pressing.

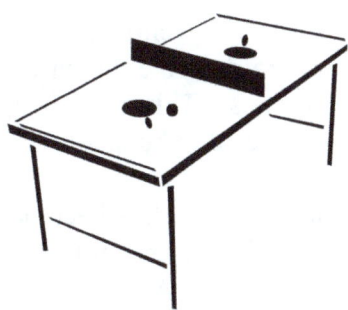

If you are considering having or adopting a baby, you should continue reading. This book will help you assess *before you conceive or adopt* whether you and your partner can have a solid parent-partnership. A critical first step for creating a great parent-partnership is to decide consciously who will be your child's other parent. Some wise grandmother was probably talking about selecting a mate when she said, "An ounce of prevention is worth of pound of cure."

If you already have a child or if a baby is on the way, you should also continue reading. This book will help ensure that you will have the strongest and most supportive relationship possible with your child's other parent.

Even if you are unsure about whether the "parent-partner" concept has anything to offer you, you should still continue reading. By the end of this book, you will hopefully agree that children receive important advantages when their parents act as good parent-partners, and that most parents can achieve a solid parent-partnership, or at least something closer to it than their present arrangement. Perhaps you will even become a proponent for changing the law so that all children might have parents who are "parent-partners."

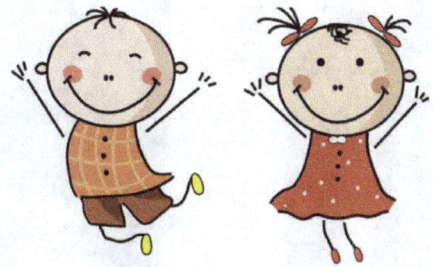

Finally, if you are curious about the ideas in the larger academic book, well, this book will introduce you to the ideas in it (specifically, point 19 at the end of this book discusses the academic book). Beware, however. This book is *not* the "Cliff Notes" or an abbreviated version of the larger book. After you read this book, do not assume that you've read *A Parent-Partner Status for American Family Law*. You haven't. But you will be on your way to understanding the importance of that bigger project.

**A Note About
the Applicability of the Parent-Partner Concept
for Same-Sex Parents and Adoptive Parents**

Regarding same-sex parents: Because most children have both a mother and a father, this book, at times, uses *gendered language* to describe the parents. Of course, it is entirely possible that a child has two mothers or two fathers. This book is applicable to same-sex families too, and the use of gendered language is not meant to be disrespectful.

Regarding adoptive parents: Because most parents become parents through childbirth, and not adoption, this book mentions pregnancy, labor, and birth much more than adoption. However, the book is applicable to adoptive families too. As soon as two people decide to adopt together, they should be acting like parent-partners.

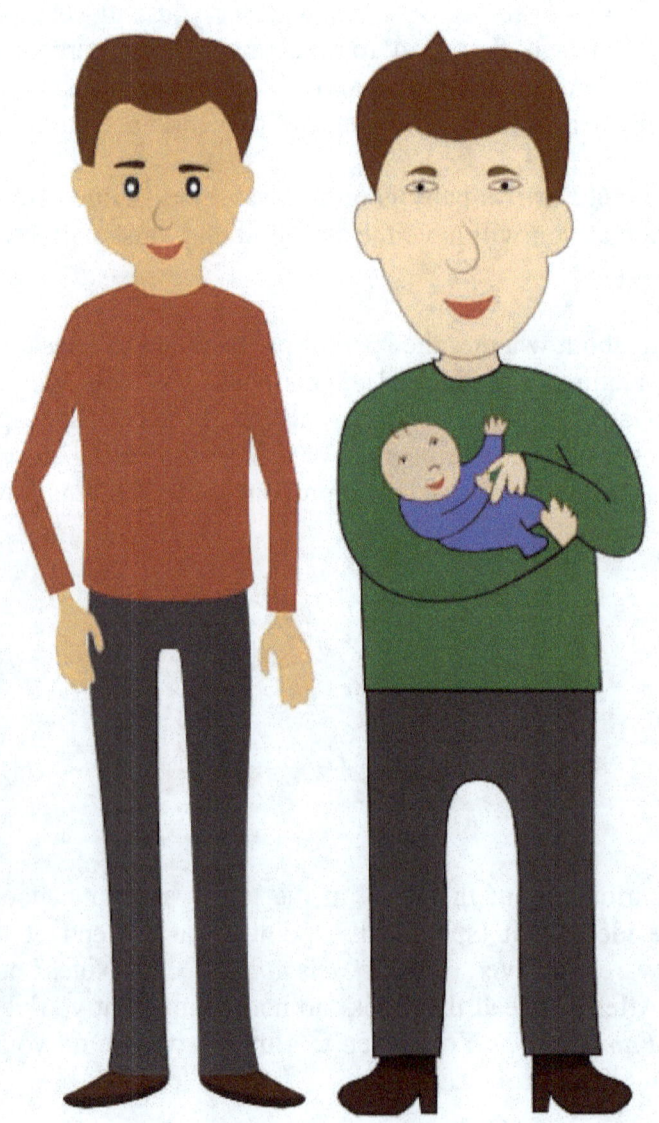

Why Would I Want to be a Parent-Partner?

One of the greatest gifts that parents can give to their child is a strong and supportive partnership with each other. (Admittedly, children might prefer an iPad or a bike, but that's besides the point.). This type of partnership should exist regardless of the other ways parents structure their relationship with each other. That means a solid parent-partnership can and should exist *in addition* to marital and romantic commitments. In fact, a good parent-partnership can and should exist even after the parents' romantic relationship ends, and even if the parents meet other romantic partners. Simply, all parents, married or not, romantic or not, should have a sound parent-partnership from the moment of their child's birth until their own death.

Of course, people can and do parent alone. Single parents can be great parents. This book is not about parenting; that is, it is not about a parent's relationship with his or her child. Nor is this book about whether people should ever become single mothers or fathers by choice. Rather, this book addresses the fact that most children from birth do have two parents who want to be involved in their children's lives. This book is about ensuring that both parents stay involved in their children's lives *by focusing on the importance of the parents' relationship to each other as a critical component for achieving that objective.*

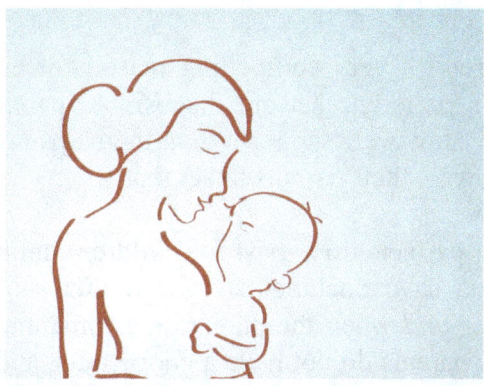

The famous basketball coach John Wooden once said, "The best thing a father can do for his children is to love their mother." That insightful comment requires a bit of updating for today's world in light of gender equality and the fact that co-parenting occurs in all sorts of relationships. Today Coach Wooden's quote should read as follows: "The best thing a parent can do for his or her child is to have a supportive partnership with the other parent."

By committing to a strong partnership with the other parent, parents can make their children's lives better. Psychologists are clear that children suffer real harm when their parents have a highly conflicted relationship with each other, that is, a relationship characterized by physical violence, psychological abuse, and/or unresolved hostility. As a result, children often become depressed, experience lower self-esteem, suffer in school, engage in anti-social behavior, and have poor relationships with their parents. Even children's moral compasses can be affected; critical traits such as empathy may never develop fully or at all. Children without empathy grow up to be unpleasant and sometimes dangerous adults.

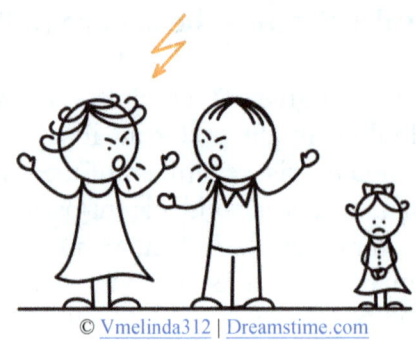

© Vmelinda312 | Dreamstime.com

Fortunately, not every bit of conflict hurts children. "Thank goodness," you might be saying, because who doesn't occasionally argue with his or her partner? Conflict is more likely to be harmful if it is frequent, intense (including physical violence and a high degree of negative hostility), child-focused, and unresolved.

However, even if parents do not have a hostile relationship, they should *strive* for a *supportive* relationship. As Dr. Kyle Pruett and Dr. Marsha Kline Pruett said in their book, *Partnership Parenting*, "Children know and deeply appreciate when parents show each other respect, positive attitudes, and affection for each other over ire – even when they disagree."

Yet children's preferences aren't a very compelling reason for encouraging adults to act in a particular way. If children's preferences were dispositive, parents would have to feed their children dessert all the time. However, supportive partnerships are important for other reasons too, not just because children want their parents to act that way.

Simply, a supportive parental partnership *is* best for children, unlike serving children ice cream at every meal. Psychologists have documented that mutual support matters *both* when the parents are no longer together *and* when the parents are romantically involved. Children lose real advantages in life if their parents do not have a cooperative and supportive partnership at all times.

How Exactly Does a Cooperative and Supportive Relationship Benefit My Child?

When parents have that type of relationship, they are more likely to enjoy parenting and find that the experience is fun. Jane Goodall once remarked (after giving birth to a son nicknamed Grub), "One thing I had learned from watching chimpanzees with their infants is that having a child should be *fun*." While ideally childrearing would always be enjoyable, it often falls short of being a blast because raising children is really hard work. However, raising a child *is likely* to be fun more of the time when you share that hard work, as well as your child's achievements and milestones, with the other parent.

In addition, a solid relationship with the other parent reduces parenting stress. Less stress makes parents better at parenting, and strengthens each parent's relationship with his or her child. Parents tend not to be at their best when they are stressed. In nature, pressure produces diamonds, but in parenting, pressure can produce parents with short tempers and other problems.

Parental cooperation and support also make the sum of the parents' efforts greater than their individual parts. Think of it this way, a peanut butter and jelly sandwich is much better than a peanut butter sandwich or jelly sandwich by itself. When both parents operate together as a team, the result is like a peanut butter and jelly sandwich. In terms of day-to-day parenting, for example, when one parent is busy and can't meet the child's needs, the other parent can jump in to do so. That interchangeability between parents benefits the child.

When the parents' romantic relationship ends, a supportive and cooperative partnership keeps both parents involved in their children's lives. Parents who were cooperative and supportive during their romantic relationship recognize more readily that both parents have value to their child and *to each other*. Therefore, they are much more likely to have a strong partnership after breakup. Without a supportive and cooperative partnership after breakup, one parent (and it is typically the father) often becomes less involved. He can even disappear altogether, as if a magician went "poof." People pull back when they are made to feel unnecessary and unwanted. This withdrawal is unfortunate for children because children with two loving parents have it twice as good as children with one.

Given that approximately 40% of children will experience their parents' divorce, and an even higher percentage will experience the breakup of their unmarried parents' relationships, parents should do everything they can *during* their romantic relationship to establish a supportive, cooperative co-parenting relationship. Supportive co-parenting early in a relationship becomes an insurance policy; it is a resource that can be drawn upon if it is ever needed. It also decreases the likelihood that the romantic relationship will end. The effect is like an auto insurance policy that could ward off auto accidents!

Parental support and cooperation have other benefits too. A great parental relationship can reduce the economic hardship associated with family breakup. Family breakup is expensive! Two places to live can cost more than one. Sometimes parents spend their money foolishly, to compensate for their hurt feelings or to show their children that they are still loved. Employment can become harder to maintain if one parent relied on the other parent's childcare to make market work possible. Unfortunately, the economic hardship from family breakup contributes to children's diminished educational and job prospects. Children who live with only one biological parent have less chance of economic mobility than their peers. But parents with a great relationship can work together to mitigate these effects.

Even apart from these benefits to parents and children, parents should act like good parent-partners because it is the right thing to do. Children deserve parents who show the level of commitment that a good parent-partnership necessitates. Simply, children deserve their parents' best effort! No parent purposefully leaves out a key ingredient when they bake a cake; why should parents leave out a key ingredient when they raise their children?

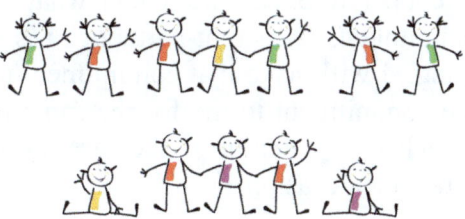

What if the Other Person Doesn't Want to be an Good Parent-Partner?

You are lucky if you are *not* asking this question. If both you and your partner are excited and ready to become good parent-partners or you two are already good parent-partners, then you can *skip this section* and move on to the next! See, a commitment to being a good parent-partner is already paying you dividends! You can skip ahead!

Yet, if the other person does not want to become a good parent-partner, then the answer to the question will depend upon your circumstances.

If you are considering having a child with such a person, think again. Actually, as you are thinking, run away from that person. Anyone who cannot commit to being a parent-partner over the long-term should not reproduce with you. Period!

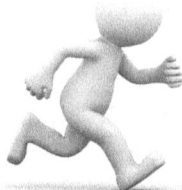

Don't be foolish and believe that the other person will come around during the pregnancy or once the child is born. Most likely, he or she will not. Sorry for the bad news, but a bit of truth today is better than a lot of heartache tomorrow. You should not gamble with your child's well-being, hoping that the other person will step up and act like a good parent-partner should.

If you are married and thinking about having a child, and the other person cannot even verbalize a commitment to being a solid parent-partner, then the gamble is similarly unacceptable. Just because you are married to someone doesn't mean you should have a child with that person. People marry for many reasons and your partner's willingness to take the plunge (especially at a time when divorce is readily available) says nothing about that person's suitability for, or commitment to, a parent-partnership. We are almost brainwashed to think the opposite, however. Who hasn't heard the nursery rhyme: "First comes love, then comes marriage, then comes baby in the baby carriage"? We need a new jingle. Perhaps it should be, "First comes love, then comes marriage, next comes a commitment to a parent-partnership, and then comes baby in the baby carriage."

If you already have a child with a person who is skeptical about the parent-partner concept and you two are on *good terms*, the other person is likely to come around. You should explain the parent-partner idea. Say something like the following: "I know you love our daughter and want her to have all possible advantages in life. Psychologists say it is best for our child if we can commit to being a supportive, cooperative team no matter what else happens. It doesn't cost a penny for us to make this commitment. A parent-partnership is supposed to benefit us too by decreasing the stress of parenting. I will make that commitment to you for our daughter's sake, and I hope you make the same commitment to me for the same reason." If there is hesitation, encourage the person to read this book. When he or she agrees to act like a good parent-partner, bring that person a gift! Celebrate the occasion!

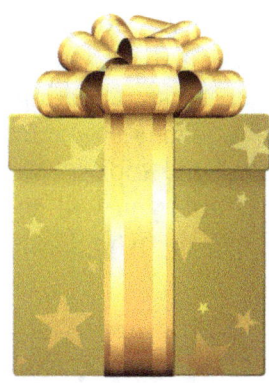

If you already have a child with your partner and the two of you are *not on good terms*, it is not impossible to develop a solid parent-partnership (assuming the other person isn't abusive or a danger to you or your child). You can try to convince the person to learn about the benefits of being parent-partners. You might text or email the person a link to this book or send this book to him or her by the old-fashioned postal service. You can ask if the other parent would see a relationship counselor with you. You can also try to create a self-fulfilling prophecy: act like a good parent-partner yourself and then reinforce with positive feedback any small steps that the other parent takes in the right direction. You should emphasize that strengthening your relationship will benefit your child.

You can also use the well-known "I-statement" to try to get the other parent to change his or her mind. The "I-statement" requires describing the problematic behavior, identifying the effects of that behavior on you, describing how that behavior makes you feel, and suggesting a solution. Here is an example: "When you ignore me in front of Billy, I get really depressed and cannot concentrate. We should learn more about the parent-partner idea so that we can be the best possible parents for Billy." Some people respond better when they hear about how their behavior affects their children. For those people, the "child-statement" would be more effective: "When you ignore me in front of Billy, Billy gets sad and sometimes cries. We should learn more about becoming parent-partners so that we can be the best possible parents for Billy."

"I-STATEMENT" OR "CHILD-STATEMENT"

Of course, if the other parent were already a good parent-partner, that parent would respond by listening, repeating what he or she heard the problem to be, empathizing, and then either respectfully agree with the solution or propose another one. In the above example, the other parent might respond, "Billy gets sad when I ignore you." Even if the other parent disagreed with some part of your "child-statement," a good parent-partner would avert conflict by saying, "I am not sure I agree, but you believe Billy is bothered by my actions. That is a good enough reason for us to learn about becoming better parent-partners." If you and your partner were already good parent-partners, a solution would likely be forthcoming because flexibility is an attribute of a good parent-partnership.

Yet if you and the other parent have unresolved hostility, the other parent may never accept the parent-partner philosophy. This can be difficult to swallow. Nonetheless, you will have improved your situation if the other person starts acting even a little more cooperatively and supportively after hearing about the philosophy's advantages for your child. And, you never know what might result from broaching the topic. Most parents want to do right by their children. If you don't ask the question, then you will never have the chance to get the answer you want. Or, to put it another way, "The baby who doesn't cry, doesn't get fed!"

The **good news** is that if you are *expecting a child and you follow the instructions* that are discussed next, you are unlikely ever to fall into this last category. That is a good thing because the last category is a frustrating place to be.

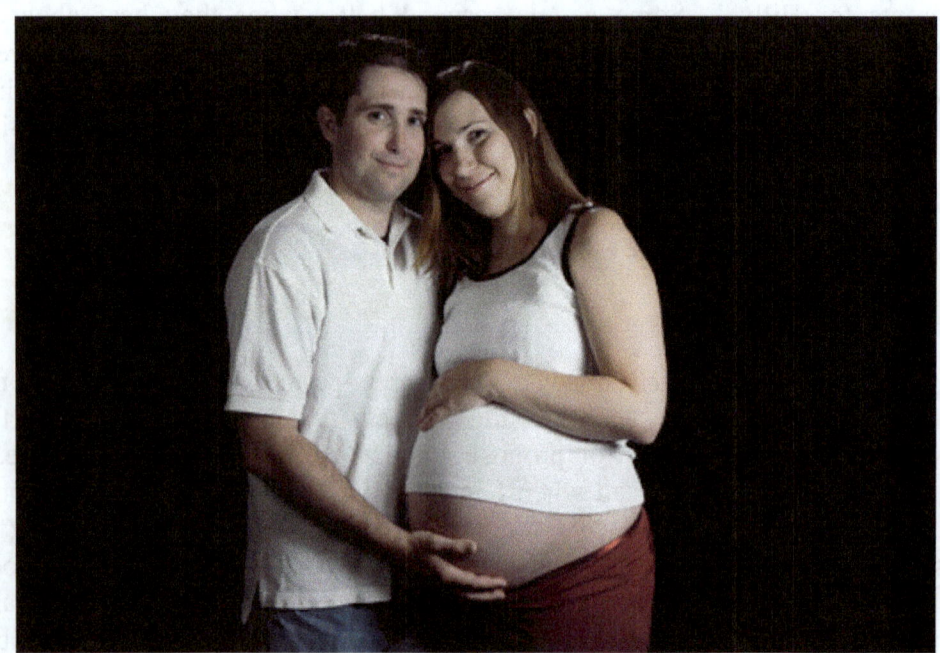

© Alexeys | Dreamstime.com

Some Steps for Becoming A Parent-Partner
(With Tips for Creating a Strong Parent-Partnership and Facts to Convince You To Do So).

1) Recognize that becoming a parent is a life-altering event, and that it will affect your relationship with your partner for the worse.

For the *worse*?

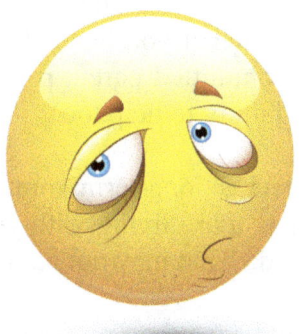

Yes, for the worse. While a new baby is wonderful and typically brings the parents great pride and joy, a new baby also strains the parents' relationship. Older couples should warn younger couples that this will happen, but they rarely do. Perhaps they are reluctant to admit that their own romantic relationships declined in quality after their children's births. Perhaps they fear people will judge them. Regardless, new parents have misconceptions about how life will be after their baby arrives because considerable silence surrounds this topic.

What is the truth? Most couples experience a decline in the quality of the romantic relationship after they transition to parenthood. This is true whether the parents are married or unmarried. After all, new parents are tired. Chores increase. Gendered patterns develop. Parenting is hard and it strains even the best of relationships.

The good news, however, is that *this outcome is not a unique experience*. Almost everyone experiences it. The other good news is that many couples come through this experience with their relationships intact. There is light at the end of the tunnel. Finally, there is still more good news: parents can minimize the strain. New parents can take a course or meet with a counselor who will help them keep the romantic relationship strong as they transition to parenthood. Therapeutic activities have been shown to maintain the quality of parents' romantic relationships.

Don't be fooled if you feel happier after your child's birth than you were during the pregnancy, especially if the pregnancy was unplanned. Parenthood may not seem quite as problematic as you imagined. You may be experiencing a blip of happiness. Unfortunately, this effect is typically temporary. Couples with unplanned pregnancies, like couples with planned pregnancies, usually find that the quality of their relationship eventually falls below the pre-pregnancy baseline even if their relationship is initially better than it was during the pregnancy.

2) Make sure that the person who might be your parent-partner will be a good parent-partner.

Warning! If you aren't enthusiastic about raising a child with your partner over the long-term, do not have unprotected sex (and don't adopt with that person either, although admittedly an adoption is a lot less likely since legal proceedings do not produce orgasms!). This warning does not mean that you should refrain from sex. Rather, this warning means that you should refrain from *unprotected* sex.

No matter how great and capable you are, and no matter how much you want a child, it is hard to raise a child on your own. It doesn't matter if you have other people in your family to help. It will still be harder than if you had a committed parent-partner *plus* those other people to help (and the other people in your partner's family to help too).

Just so you know, it is harder to meet a long-term romantic partner if you come into the relationship with a child, especially if you are living with your child. Do not assume that you will meet someone after you have a child. That may not happen.

Most important, since your child will not have the same advantages in life as other children with two parents who act as good parent-partners, it is *wrong* to conceive when you think at the outset that your child might not have two parents who are committed to parenting together supportively for the long-term. "Wrong" is an intentionally strong word.

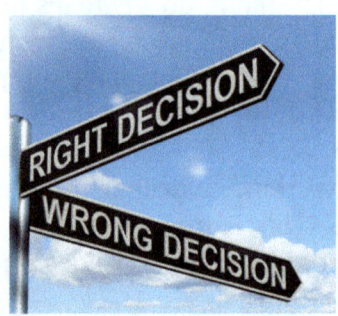

The only exception may be a "single parent by choice" (SPC). A SPC is someone who adopts alone or uses a sperm donor or surrogate to conceive. Most SPCs are economically privileged so their children are not economically disadvantaged from being raised by a single parent, and SPCs typically establish support networks that are ready and willing to help. So for SPCs, "unwise" might be a more appropriate word than "wrong." While SPCs can and do raise children well, they are the first to admit that it is easier to do so when there are two parents.

What the foregoing means is that if you are considering conception with a partner, be choosey! If your partner or your relationship has problems, think twice about having unprotected sex. Better yet, think twice and then **don't** have unprotected sex with that person. While most people do not have a baby to improve a problematic relationship or to bring out the best in a troubled partner, some people do. These optimists believe that a baby will change their partners or relationships for the better. These optimists are operating under a dangerous delusion. It is more likely that the exact opposite will happen: a baby will make things worse.

If someone is generally rude, mean, inflexible, or a jerk to the outside world (to parents, teachers, friends, or others), that person is unlikely to be different in his or her relationship with a parent-partner. At some point, those traits are likely to emerge in the parent-partnership. Ask yourself, "Can I see raising a child with this person for at least the next 18 years?"

If someone is violent, drug addicted, an alcoholic, or involved in crime, that person is engaging in behavior that is inconsistent with being a good parent-partner. Those sorts of behaviors will put you and your child's safety at risk. A good parent-partner, one who is fond of his or her partner, would not put the partner's safety at risk. Before you have a baby with such a person, let that person clean up his or her act, and then stay clean for at least a couple of years. Remember, a baby can bring stress, and stress can trigger a reoccurrence of bad habits.

✔**Fact:** Having a child usually will *not* make a bad relationship better.

✔**Fact:** Having a child usually will *not* make a bad partner better.

Do **NOT** roll the dice!

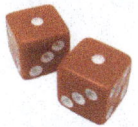

If you want to make your romantic relationship stronger, try adopting a dog and see how that goes.

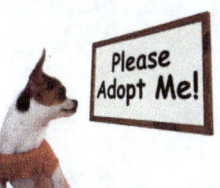

Seriously, you should try something besides having a baby. Here are some other ideas: try starting a business together, moving in together, or getting married. All of these options are reversible. You can divorce your spouse if it doesn't work out, but once you have a baby with someone you have a life-long connection. If you are seeking a unique experience to bring you two closer together, consider hiking the Pacific Crest trail. By the end of the 2,600-mile hike, you'll have a better idea of whether or not your partner is baby-making material.

If you are unsure what qualities you should be seeking in a solid parent-partner, you will be able to identify those qualities after you read point 5 below. As you will soon discover, you need to make sure that your partner exhibits "f.f.a.t.e." *before* you conceive. Be on the lookout for the meaning of "f.f.a.t.e." It is essential to a successful parent-partnership!

3) Make sure that you know how to prevent pregnancy and then prevent it until you have a worthy parent-partner.

What do you call a woman who doesn't use birth control effectively? A mother.

And what do you call a man who doesn't use birth control effectively? A father.

Don't gamble with your choice of a partner and don't gamble with your fertility either!

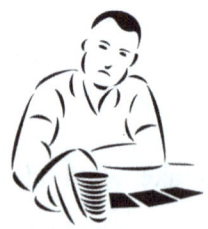

<u>**A little information about birth control:**</u>

If 100 people use only the diaphragm, 16 will get pregnant.

If 100 people use only a condom, 15 will get pregnant.

If 100 people use only the pill, 8 will get pregnant.

If 100 people use only a patch, 1 will get pregnant.

If 100 people use only an IUD, 1 will get pregnant.

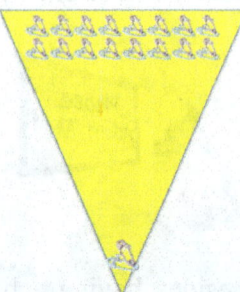

If you don't use contraceptives, or use them only sometimes, a pregnancy is very likely to occur. If 100 women have unprotected sex, 6 to 30 will get pregnant, depending upon the time of the month when intercourse occurs.

Sometimes people are uninformed about the usefulness of contraception. Some people believe that when it is time for the woman to get pregnant, she will get pregnant no matter what. That is nonsense. Pregnancy is largely preventable. We live at a time of remarkable scientific achievement. Scientists have figured out how to put a person on the moon. They have eradicated diseases like smallpox. They have developed an Internet that instantly connects people around the globe. Do not doubt that scientists have figured out how to prevent pregnancy.

What are duplicative precautions? It's when two types of birth control are used.

We all know that if something is important, it makes sense to have an extra precaution or a back-up plan. For example, you might set two alarm clocks when you need to wake up for an important appointment, event, or trip.

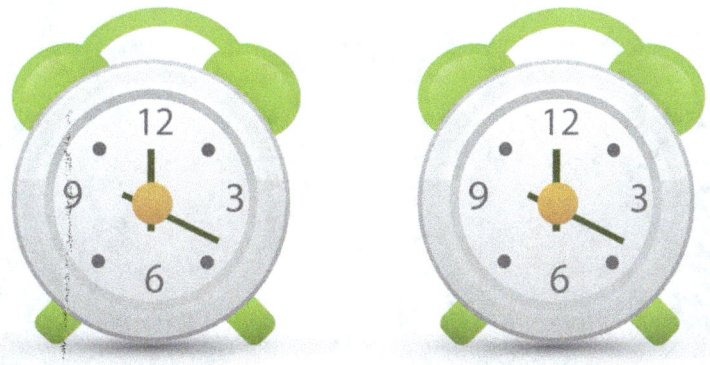

If you and your partner want to avoid a pregnancy, use two types of birth control. *Take duplicative precautions*.

If that recommendation is too expensive or troublesome, be sure to use the most effective type of birth control: a patch or an IUD.

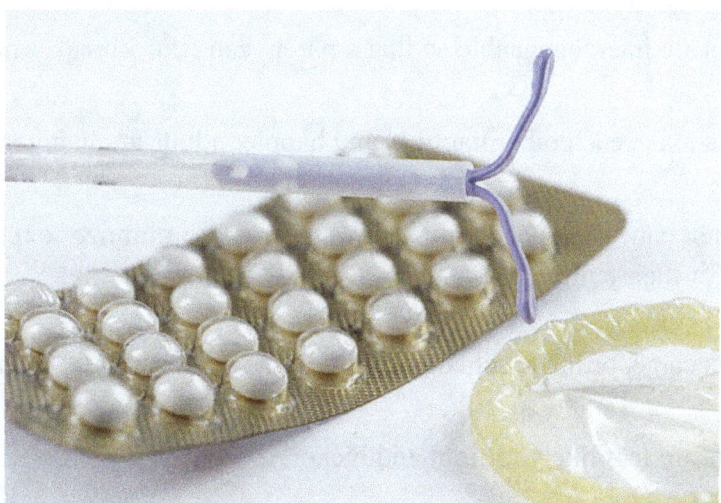

© Jpcprod | Dreamstime.com

The morning-after pill, also known by various names such as Plan B or Next Choice, is also an option. This emergency contraceptive is the drug levonorgestrel. It is 95% effective if the woman takes it within 24 hours after sex. It is 88% effective if she takes it within 72 hours. It is available over the counter; that is, you can get it without a prescription. Talk to the pharmacist about any other medication or supplements the woman is taking. But please *do not use* an emergency contraceptive as a form of birth control. If you use it as your only method of birth control for an entire year, you'll have a 20% chance of getting pregnant. Also, be aware that the morning-after pill may not work as well for people who weigh over 165 pounds.

4) Acknowledge the following truth and then share the information with your partner: Kids do best when their parents' relationship is cooperative and supportive.

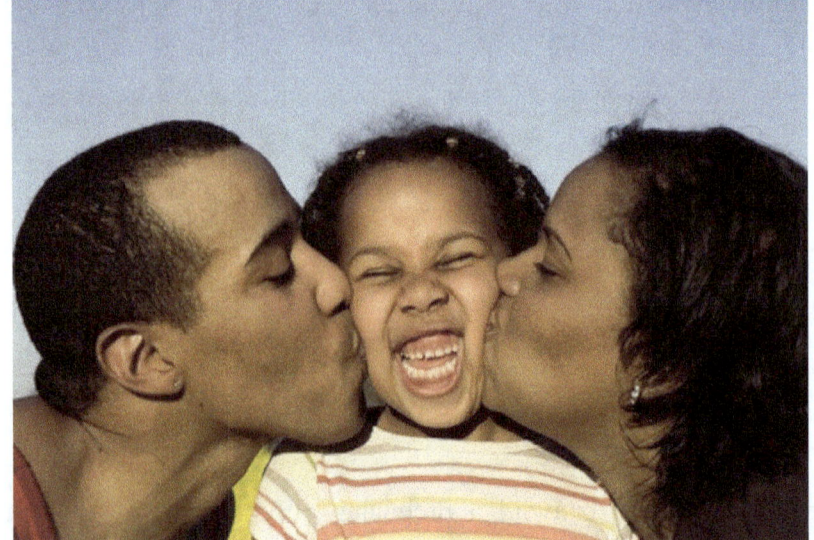
© Htuller | Dreamstime.com

As mentioned above, psychologists have documented that children do best when their parents have a supportive partnership. The benefits come in many forms.

✔Supportive parents are interchangeable so that a parent can take a break when stressed.

✔Supportive parents make each other happier, and happier adults are happier parents.

✔Supportive parents can share economic resources and minimize expenses to maximize financial resources for their child.

✔Supportive parents can coordinate schedules to increase opportunities for their child.

✔Supportive parents are less likely to fight and bicker.

✔Supportive parents are less likely to see their romantic relationships end.

✔Supportive parents who split up are much more likely to co-parent successfully.

Here is a jingle to help you recall this critical message. It is sung to the tune of Twinkle, Twinkle Little Star: "Parent-Partner, of my kid, How I wonder what we did. Raised a child so wonderful, Supported each other through it all. Parent-Partner of my kid. Thank you friend for what we did."

5) Live a life consistent with the values reflected in the parent-partner concept.

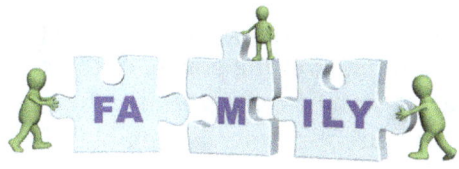

© Frenta | Dreamstime.com

Society at present has very few expectations for parents that have a child in common. That doesn't mean that you should have few expectations for your own relationship.

First, you should consider your parent-partnership to be a family relationship. Society expects family members to show each other a certain amount of affection, consideration, concern, sacrifice, fairness, respect, acceptance, support, and responsibility. You and your parent-partner will have a family relationship regardless of whether you two are married or unmarried, or your romantic relationship ends. In fact, it is *false* to think that parent-partners who breakup no longer have "a relationship" with each other. They still have a *family* relationship. Their child makes them a family forever.

Parents with a child in common are family; yet, they are also a specific type of family. They are parent-partners. This type of family relationship entails additional expectations. After all, society expects different behavior from siblings than from spouses. While society currently lacks clear expectations for parent-partners, we can identify what society's expectations should be and then hold parents (and ourselves) accountable for meeting them.

Studies reveal that *successful co-parents exhibit five particular qualities* after breakup. These five qualities make parents resilient and able to work together. Society should expect parent-partners to exhibit these five qualities from the get-go. You should look for these five qualities in a parent-partner, you should exhibit these five qualities to your parent-partner, and you should expect your parent-partner to show you these qualities.

These are the f.f.a.t.e. qualities that were mentioned earlier in point 2. If you have been looking for them, here they are.

Fondness: Good parent-partners are fond of each other. When you think about the other parent, you should be glad that you have a connection. What are the things about the other person that make you fond of him or her? Identify what those qualities are and keep them foremost in your mind. Is it because the other person is nice, smart, strong, devoted, capable, talented, a hard worker, etc.? Perhaps you are fond of the other person's sense of humor; perhaps he or she is funny and could really spice up this book! Once you identify those qualities, share your appreciation of those qualities with your parent-partner. Say, for example, "I really like that you are so talented." After all, everyone loves a compliment.

By the way, I really appreciate that you've gotten this far in the book. Thank you. You are obviously someone who cares about the well-being of children. Hopefully, my little bit of flattery proves the point that compliments feel good, even between strangers!

Flexibility: A good parent-partner recognizes that "give and take" is essential for a good relationship, and then exhibits flexibility with his or her partner. Sometimes one person will give, and at times the other parent will give. The other parent's giving may not be an immediate reaction to the first parent's giving, but over the course of the relationship there should be a give and take. Flexibility makes life go so much more easily. In essence, flexibility is the grease on the wheels of life. Every time a parent-partner is flexible, that parent-partner strengthens the parent-partnership.

Acceptance: Parent-partners accept those parts of the other parent that can't be changed. Parent-partners are not clones of each other. Parent-partners differ from each other in countless ways. As the great philosopher Dr. Suess once wrote, "There is no one alive that is you-er than you." While some couples tend to become more like each other over time (isn't that an interesting phenomenon?), important differences will always remain. Accept those differences even if you are not fond of those differences. For example, if your partner is an unrepentant slob, accept it and try to recognize its advantages. Supposedly, out of chaos comes creativity, so perhaps the mess will lead to a cure for cancer or to the invention of a flying car. Of course, your parent-partner should similarly accept all of your qualities that you cannot (or will not) change, including your obsession with cleanliness.

Togetherness: All of the major co-parenting challenges should be tackled together. This orientation makes the challenges easier to resolve. Imagine, for example, that one parent gets a great job offer in another city. Imagine the offer is to become the CEO of Google, the lead in a new Andrew Lloyd Webber musical, or the head coach for the number-one-ranked college basketball team. What fabulous opportunities! Regardless of whether the couple is romantically involved or not, any job opportunity in another city can cause real strain between parent-partners (even a job that is not nearly so attractive as those mentioned above). The couple must work together to assess the options, decide which is the best option for their child, and then achieve that option or minimize the disadvantages from another chosen option. To see how this works, assume that the parents in this example are no longer romantically involved. There are three options, although most couples only consider the first two. First, the parent with the job offer can leave. Second, the parent with the job offer can stay. Third, the parent with the job offer can leave and the other parent can follow. When parents work together to overcome co-parenting challenges, they have more opportunities to find solutions.

Togetherness also means that couples stand united before their child on the important issues. So, for example, when the parent with the job offer decides to move and the other parent decides to stay, the parents should unite in the message about that decision. They both need to tell the child how they will make things work best for the child in light of the change.

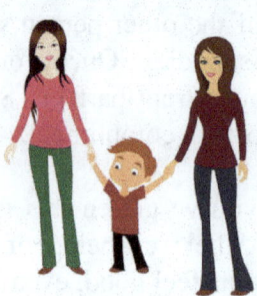

Empathy: Life is hard and it often involves countless ups and downs. Even day-to-day living can be hard, especially when conditions are less than ideal. Money may be short, jobs may be less than exciting, friends or family may have problems, and our own problems may cause us to struggle. Sometimes a parent-partner can help solve some of these problems, but often not. What a parent-partner can always do, however, is care. Caring involves listening as well as expressing sympathy and concern about the obstacles in the other parent's life.

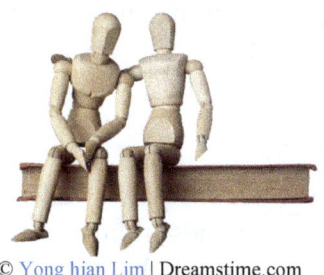
© Yong hian Lim | Dreamstime.com

If you find someone with all five of the above qualities, he or she is likely to be a good parent-partner. You can remember these five qualities because the first letter of each quality spells out the word **f.f.a.t.e** (albeit with two fs): **f**ondness, **f**lexibility, **a**cceptance, **t**ogetherness, and **e**mpathy. Once two people have a child together, **f.f.a.t.e.** connects them.

✔**Fact:** Parents are more likely to have a long-lasting romantic relationship with each other if they focus on the positives (that is, their progress and growth as a team) rather than on the negatives, including the uncertainty that they may have about their romantic relationship's future.

✔**Tip:** Think of your relationship as getting better and better. While there may be challenges, there are undoubtedly some accomplishments too. Make a conscious decision to have a healthy, loving relationship and then *work* to make your relationship better.

Celebrate your relationship's achievements as often as possible. If you've been together a certain number of months or years, celebrate! If you've managed to stay together during the first year of your child's life, celebrate! If your partner has overcome a personal challenge, such as substance abuse, celebrate! If your partner recently exhibited one of the traits that you admire, celebrate! If your partner accomplished anything worth praising (and there is usually *something* to praise), compliment him or her! Celebrate the positives in your parent-partner and your parent-partnership. Celebrations will make your relationship stronger.

6) Regardless of whether you are married or unmarried, start acting as parent-partners from the moment the pregnancy begins, if not earlier.

A solid parent-partnership is not just about parenting well together. It is also about having a supportive relationship overall. It is the sort of relationship that exists between good friends.

It is hard, if not impossible, to work as a co-parenting team if one person treats the other parent as a jerk, as incompetent, or as unworthy of respect. While you can't control how your parent-partner acts toward you, you can control how you act toward your parent-partner. Treat your parent-partner as a good friend.

It sometimes seems like magic, but when one party puts in the effort and treats the other person well, then the other person typically responds in kind. Ralph Waldo Emerson once said, "The only way to have a friend is to be one." Similarly, the only way to have a good parent-partner is to be one.

Unsolicited acts of kindness can go a long way in building a great partnership. Do something nice for your partner "just because." Act excited to see him or her when he or she walks in the room (try imitating a dog who is happy to see his or her owner). Sit by your parent-partner; don't sit on the other side of the room. Body language says a lot. Lavish gifts on your parent-partner. They can be as simple as homemade cards or daisies picked from the side of the road.

People often live up to your views of them. If you treat your parent-partner as a special individual, he or she is likely to become that special individual.

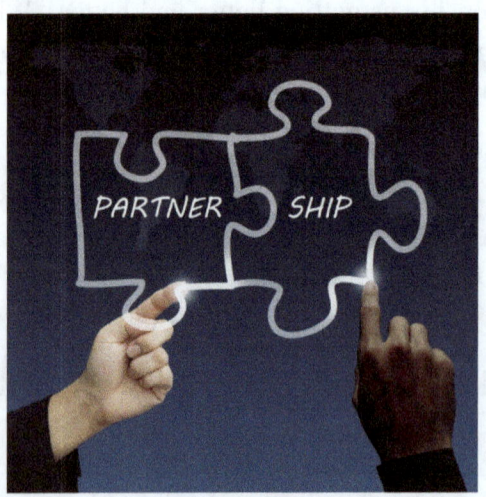

The time to start with a supportive friendship is as *early* as possible. Ideally, that is *before* you start having sex. After all, even the best contraceptives sometimes fail. In heterosexual couples, there is *always* a risk that two lovers will end up as parent-partners (assuming both parties are fertile). Lovers should talk about what will happen if a pregnancy occurs. Communicating with your partner about the prospect of becoming parent-partners is respectful. It allows you both to make an informed decision together about how to minimize the risk and whether the remaining risk is worth it.

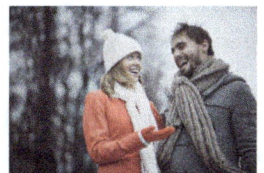

Certainly, when you are *planning to* become parents or when you realize a baby is coming, you need to be acting like good parent-partners.

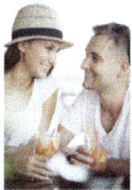

✓**Fact:** People can (and should) act as parent-partners from the moment of conception.

✓**Fact:** Every stage of your relationship builds upon the prior stage. A long-lasting partnership is best assured when each stage of your relationship is a partnership between good friends.

Pregnant Women: Let your partner into the pregnancy experience as much as possible from conception. Unless you let your partner share your experience, your partner won't have the parenthood experience until the baby is born. You have a tremendous opportunity to set the tone for a supportive, cooperative partnership. Let your partner talk to the baby. Invite your partner to your doctor appointments. Consider ways that you both might gain experience with babies, such as by visiting couples with newborns or reading books on pregnancy together. Let your partner tell others that you are pregnant and that he is the other parent. Start identifying your partner as your "parent-partner." Call your partner your "parent-partner." Simply, start treating your partner as the parent-partner that you want that person to become.

Men (or women in lesbian couples): A supportive partner starts exhibiting support immediately. The pregnancy is the easiest period during which to do so because the baby isn't there yet to make his or her own demands. Engage in unanticipated acts of kindness. For example, make her a lunch to take to work in order to show her that you care about her nutrition and the baby's health. Ask her, "Can I make you more comfortable while you are carrying our baby?" Offer her a five-minute backrub. Refer to her as your parent-partner. Consider taking classes or getting information from friends or family about caring for an infant in order to show her that you are excited and ready to parent. Be proud: publicly acknowledge your appreciation for the mother. The more you treat her like a parent-partner from the get-go, the more she will be willing to "open the gate" to let you into the pregnancy experience.

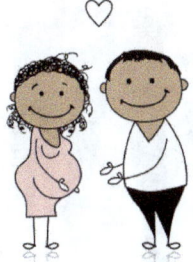

© Kydriashka | Dreamstime.com

7) Continue acting like parent-partners throughout labor and delivery.

Ninety percent (90%) of fathers are in the delivery room these days. Isn't that wonderful? Sure, childbirth can be a bit untidy, but it is nature's mess. Overall, the experience is nothing short of miraculous. It can bring a couple closer together and set the stage for a new "triangulated" relationship between the parents and their child. And yes, that new triangulated relationship will undoubtedly involve more of nature's mess, at least from the newest member.

Unfortunately, labor and delivery can also have the opposite effect on a relationship, however: the experience can start unraveling the parents' romantic relationship.

Pregnant Women: Labor and delivery are important events and you should do everything possible to encourage your partner to attend. Set aside your modesty. Childbirth is not a beauty pageant.

Dads (or supporting partners in lesbian couples): Labor and delivery are stressful and often painful events for the mom, and you must respect her choices during labor and delivery — even if she excludes you from the room. This is the time to be *super* helpful; do *whatever* she wants. If you show unqualified support for her during labor and delivery, your parent-partner is going to trust your ability to comfort and fortify her during other experiences that are not nearly as taxing.

Pregnant Women and Supporting Partners: It really helps to talk about labor and delivery *before* they occur. Programs that teach partners to be breathing coaches are useful, but these programs do not replace the detailed planning that couples should do for the labor and delivery experience. The goal is to figure out how to support each other during the big event. Since the pregnant woman is not expected to be as helpful to her partner during labor and delivery as the partner should be to her (for obvious reasons), the pregnant woman should, to the extent possible, anticipate her own needs ahead of time and share that information with her partner. That is one way that she can help her partner.

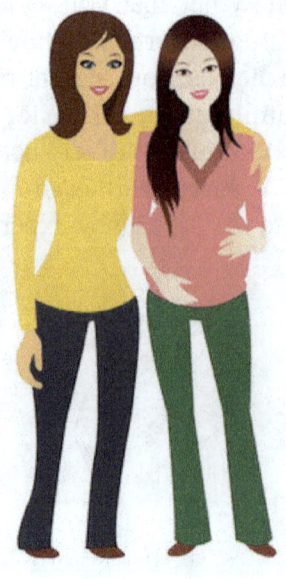

Pregnant Women: Think about your likely needs and tell them to your partner. Will you want your partner to sing? Rub your back? Film the event? Deliver popsicles? Bring your favorite pillow? Send out a text message when the baby is born? Ask your partner to take responsibility for specific tasks so that your partner feels included and useful. Assure your partner that if you become crude and curse, become mean, or become silent during the labor and delivery, your behavior isn't meant to show disrespect. Similarly, tell your partner that you may change your mind about all of the tasks that you assigned earlier (or didn't assign, but will now want). Prepare your partner. Explain ahead of time that unpredictability is common, and that hormones and pain can dictate a woman's behavior during childbirth. Also, warn your partner that the hospital staff may not treat him or her as part of the team, but that you view your partner as part of the team and are very glad that he or she will be there with you.

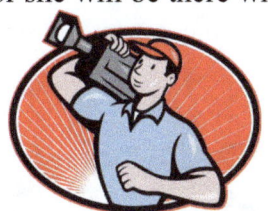

Dads (or supporting partners in lesbian couples): Create a plan before labor and delivery about how you will be helpful. Listen to what your partner tells you that she will need. However, also use your ingenuity to anticipate her needs. Should you bring a cooler with popsicles just in case she changes her mind and wants one? Can you bring her gifts to open on the hour in order to make the time go faster and to show her that you care enough to wrap many small trinkets for her distraction? Can you write a love song for her or the baby? How about making the baby a time capsule to be opened in 18 years, and showing its contents to your partner during labor?

Fathers commonly feel excluded and unhelpful at labor and delivery, especially as they are often unable to lessen the mother's pain. Some fathers have equated the experience with torture. Yes, torture. Anticipate these possibilities and do not let them overwhelm you. Know that your presence means a lot to your partner regardless of what is happening in the labor and delivery room. Your support will show her that she can count on you. It will also set the stage for what is to come later in your partnership.

Note for Gay Men: These labor and delivery tips may also apply to gay men who are using a surrogate to help create their family. Regardless of whether the surrogate wants your company, your partner certainly does. Comfort and support each other as your surrogate is in labor.

Warning! Labor and delivery can cause expectant parents to start growing apart. Don't let that happen to you. Let it be a time when you stay strong and even grow closer together.

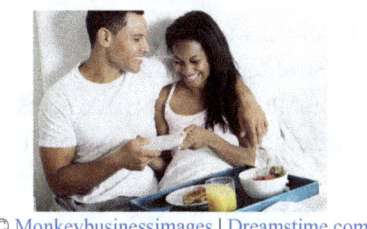

© Monkeybusinessimages | Dreamstime.com

8) Celebrate your parent-partner relationship at its outset.

Celebrations are part of life, especially for significant events like marriages and births. Both a ceremony and a party typically accompany entry into marriage. Baby showers are often hosted in anticipation of a child's birth. A christening, bris, or aqiqah may follow after the child's birth, depending on the parents' religion.

It is important for new parents to celebrate their new parent-partnership too. A parent-partnership is a significant relationship created by a life-changing event: the arrival of the baby. A celebration will cement the parents' commitment to act as a cooperative and supportive team throughout their child's youth. Friends and family should be invited to witness the parents' commitment. Their presence reinforces the parents' promises to make their parent-partnership succeed.

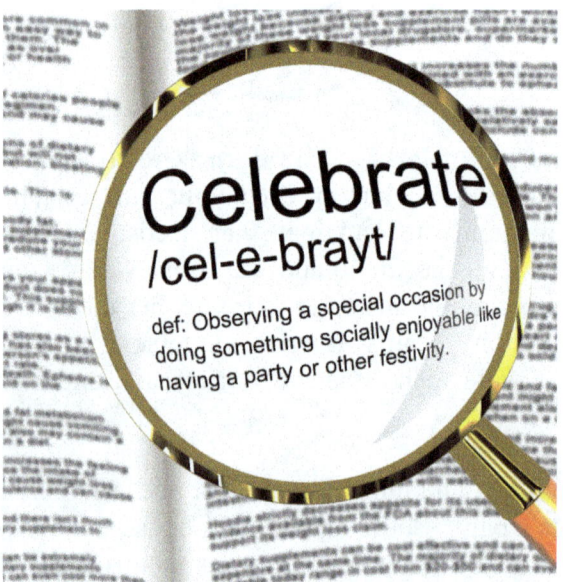

There is no right way or wrong way to celebrate. Festivities can occur before the child's birth or within a short time afterwards. The focus of this celebration is on the parents' relationship with each other, although it can certainly accompany events focused on the baby.

The government doesn't require this celebration, so no particular person needs to lead the ceremony. Parents can do it themselves, but asking a third party to assist adds a nice bit of formality to the occasion. You can ask a religious leader, a dear friend, or a family member to say a few words.

Nor is there a requirement that the words spoken by the official or exchanged between the parents have to be anything in particular. Parents should just acknowledge that they will have a supportive partnership in order to ensure that their child has all possible advantages in life. The official might want to remind the parties of those qualities that good parent-partners exhibit: fondness, flexibility, acceptance, togetherness, and empathy (see point 5 above for more on f.f.a.t.e.). If the parents have entered a written agreement (see point 15 below), the official may want to share publicly the couple's specific promises.

It would be appropriate for guests to bring gifts. After all, people give wedding gifts to a couple that may soon divorce. Approximately 20% percent of marriages end within five years, and guests often joke about wanting their gifts returned. In contrast, parents who are celebrating their parent-partnership acknowledge an enduring bond regardless of their future romantic relationship. A gift signals that the gift giver believes the couple is doing something valuable. Gifts may also encourage a couple to have the celebration ceremony (in order to get the gifts). Although this may seem unsavory, it isn't. The celebration will still help the parents reinforce their commitment to each other, and this is the very point of the event.

Couples may not want gifts, and they can certainly discourage them. Or a couple may encourage useful gifts. For instance, new parents might write on the invitation, "Please do not bring gifts, except for offers of babysitting." Most new parents would welcome cash. Money could help them pay for the relationship-work classes that are so beneficial (see point 9 next). Some parents might encourage well-wishers to contribute to a particular organization instead of giving the couple a gift directly, such as an organization that offers free relationship work to low-income couples.

It is worth emphasizing that the celebration ceremony can be as simple or as fancy as a couple wants. For recently married couples, the expense of the wedding will probably make another big event unlikely. For unmarried couples, plans to wed later may necessitate a simple celebration. For all couples, economic hardship or different priorities (such as saving for the baby's college education) may suggest that a low- or no-cost celebration is best. A low- or no-cost party can certainly be a wonderful event, too.

✔ **Tip:** Send the invitations by email or tell people in person. Host the party at a park. Ask a trusted friend to conduct the ceremony and provide recorded music for dancing. If food is desired, make it a potluck!

However a couple decides to celebrate will be absolutely fine, so long as the couple does celebrate!

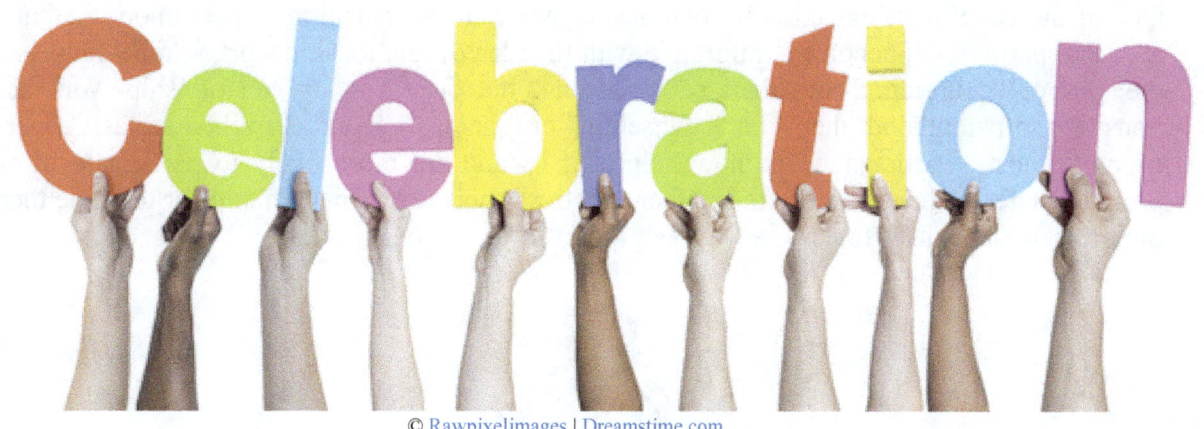

© Rawpixelimages | Dreamstime.com

9) Engage in relationship work with your partner during the transition to parenthood.

The research is clear: the quality of a couple's relationship declines during their transition to parenthood. Try your own study. Ask your parents, "Hey, did your romantic relationship go down the tubes when I was born?" If your parents are being honest, they will say that your birth caused them trouble, at least for the first few years. If you were a second child, your parents may not blame you because your older sibling may have already harmed their romantic relationship. See, there are some advantages of being the second child.

Psychologists and other professionals have developed programs that help parents keep their relationships strong. These programs are designed to be fun. They typically include information on how to support each other, communicate well, overcome hardship, keep the spark alive, etc.

These programs are *preventative*. Attending such a program does NOT mean that a relationship has failed or is failing. Rather, these programs keep good relationships going strong. They are the equivalent of stretching before exercise. They help prevent injury.

These programs are not parenting classes, but focus instead on the parents' relationship to each other. Sometimes parenting classes include this emphasis, but not always. Look for workshops or group sessions run by relationship counselors. Workshops and classes will allow you to make new friends in the process because other expectant couples will be there as well. In fact, you and some of these other couples may become lifelong friends. Alternatively, you can schedule private couple sessions with a therapist who can coach you and your partner through this difficult time. Or check with the government for free or low-cost relationship programs funded under the Healthy Marriage Initiative and Responsible Fatherhood Initiative. Try this Web site for a program near you: www.twoofus.org/area/index.aspx.

Many Web sites offer couples free advice. The U.S. government sponsors the Web site just mentioned, www.TwoOfUs.org. You should check it out. It contains some good information. While Web resources are helpful, they do not replace a more active, live experience.

One of the benefits of engaging in relationship work at the transition to parenthood is that you and your partner will become comfortable with the idea of relationship work. Some couples find the idea of "counseling" or "therapy" terrifying, but once they try relationship work at the transition to parenthood, they find "counseling" or "therapy" about as frightening as Casper the friendly ghost. Participants see how helpful it is, and are more likely to participate in other programs later in their relationships, either to refresh their parent-partnerships or to guide them if their relationships later falter.

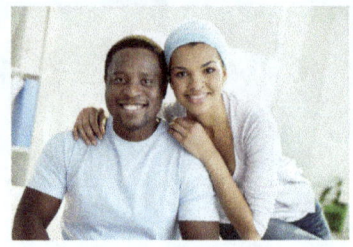

10) Step up the parent-partnership when the baby comes home.

Both parents should be involved in caring for the baby from the very beginning. Both parents are wired to do so. Moms have no unique ability to rock a baby to sleep or change a diaper. While men can't breastfeed, that is only one task among many.

There are four important reasons why both parents need to be involved in the baby's care.

First, being actively involved in your child's care *makes you a better parent-partner*. Empathy is a trait that strengthens relationships. Empathy is the ability to share the feelings of the other person. Empathy is the most genuine when you have walked in the other person's shoes. For example, a father who has never experienced exhaustion from the 3:00 a.m. feeding might have a hard time empathizing with the cranky mother. However, if the father wakes up every night at 3:00 a.m. to deliver the baby to the mother for the feeding, then he is likely to understand her feelings. Empathy grounded in experience will go far in soothing tension.

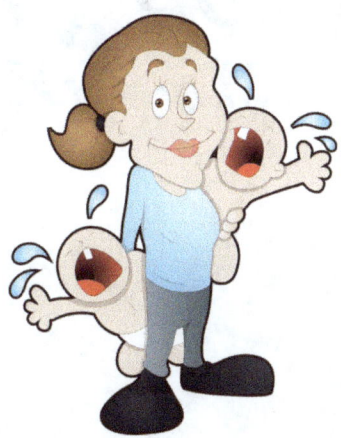

Second, being actively involved in your child's care *makes you a better parent*. People parent in different ways. Some engage in more hands-on care. Others participate more in paid employment to support the child financially. Both of these jobs are critical and there is no right way to divide the labor between the parents. Long gone are the days when women performed the hands-on care and men earned the income. Most parents today are involved in both activities. So long as the parents are both working hard to benefit their child, then each parent should be commended. However, unless both parents try hands-on parenting, the parents may not be able to assess who is better at it, enjoys it more, etc. That information is important in case one parent has to do more of the caregiving.

Moreover, very young children have a limited understanding of their parents' roles. When a parent goes away to work, the baby doesn't know where the parent is going, why the parent is leaving, or how that parent's absence benefits him or her. All the baby knows is that the parent is gone. Young children, in fact, frequently want their parents to stay home with them all day and play. Remember Kevin, the child of character Gil Buckman in *Parenthood*? He told his goofy but enthusiastic father that he wanted to work with him when he grew up so that they could spend all their time together. Children want their parents around. From the child's perspective, more hands-on care by a parent is better.

How can a parent "do diapers" when the parent has a job that takes him or her outside the home? After all, the parent can't be in two places at once. Well, that is true, but most jobs do not eat up all 24 hours in a day. There is usually some time available before and after work. A parent who works outside the house might have to forego personal and leisure time in order to spend more time with the child. Or, a parent might have to change leisure activities so that the child can participate too. Going to the gym alone may no longer be an option; jogging while pushing an infant stroller may become a necessity. A workout may now involve rebounding basketballs for your toddler. While it is not essential that both parents spend an equal amount of time caregiving, it is essential that both parents are actively involved in caregiving.

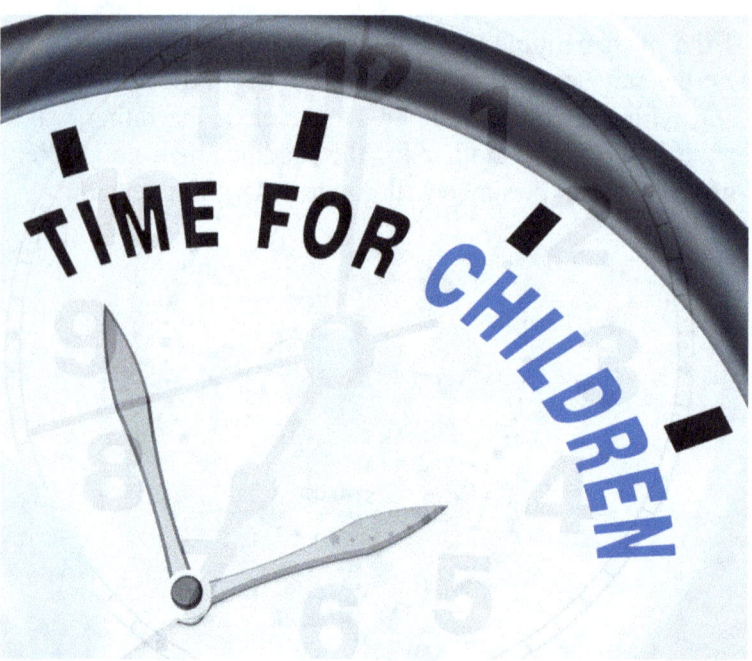

Third, being actively involved in your child's care *decreases the likelihood that you and your parent-partner will end your romantic relationship*. This point isn't based on any data, but just common sense. When both parents are actively involved in their child's care, they often work harder to maintain their romantic relationship because they want to have daily contact with their child. These parents also recognize the importance of the other parent to their child and to themselves. Women have reported that they feel particularly loved by their partners when their partners care for their children. Women may have this feeling because Mother Nature wants mothers to encourage these types of fathers to stay around.

Fourth, being actively involved in your child's care *makes it more likely that you and your parent-partner will share parenting if your romantic relationship ever ends*. Children benefit from the continued involvement of both parents in their lives after the parents split up. Children also benefit when the parents agree to share parenting without a protracted court battle. The surest way to achieve shared parenting that works well after dissolution is for parents to have shared parenting during the romantic relationship. Then both parents clearly see the advantages of having two involved parents, both for their child and for themselves. Each parent also knows that the other parent is competent and can handle the parenting tasks alone.

11) Make sure that the parent-partnership is fair.

Caregiving is not always going to be divided equally between the parents. Many couples do not split caregiving 50-50 because of work demands, practical issues, or preferences. Sometimes caregiving appears more balanced when one looks at the big picture. For example, while one parent may be doing the majority of caregiving in a particular week, month, or even year, the parents' arrangement may be fair over a longer period of time, such as over a two- or three-year period. However, lopsidedness may exist and it is okay so long as the parents have agreed to a fair arrangement. Good parent-partnerships are fair relationships.

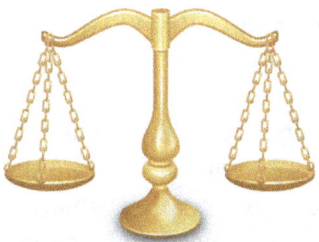

What is a "fair" arrangement differs by couple.

For married couples, a lopsided arrangement is usually made fair because the parents share economic resources. Married parents typically share the income earned by the primary breadwinner. At divorce, judges will count the caregiver's labor as a valuable contribution to the couple's acquisition of property, and will award the caregiver a fair share of it.

However, unfairness can creep into parent-partnerships. Unmarried parents (especially if they are not cohabiting) and divorced parents may find that their arrangements are unfair. One parent may perform far more of the caregiving, but the parties may not share economic resources. The primary caregiver will not have a claim to the other parent's property. This arrangement can be unfair to the primary caregiver because caregiving often produces real economic disadvantages. The need for a flexible schedule, the need for part-time work, or the need to stop and start work to accommodate caregiving can all reduce a caregiver's earnings. Data reveal that even if the primary caregiver is working full-time, caregiving can impact that parent's income over the long-term. In contrast, the parent who does less of the caregiving receives a real economic benefit. He or she has free time to earn more money or to enjoy more leisure.

Freeloading occurs when one parent does more of the caregiving, and the other parent reaps the benefits but gives nothing adequate in return. Freeloading is mooching. In Yiddish, the freeloader is called a schnorrer, which rhymes with horror (appropriately so).

Sometimes the parent who is doing the majority of the caregiving doesn't want anything in return because he or she is giving a gift of his or her labor to the other parent. But usually both parents want to feel like they are getting something equivalent from the relationship.

To be clear, child support does not include an amount to cover the value of the caregiver's labor or the hidden costs that caregiving imposes on the caregiver.

If the parents do not share caregiving 50-50, what is fair compensation for the caregiver? An outsider cannot really answer that question, especially without knowing all of the facts. Instead, the parents should answer that question themselves.

In discussing what is fair, the parents should consider several factors. First, what is the extent of the lopsidedness? Are both parents working, either at home or in the market, to benefit the child? Does one parent seem to have a lot more leisure? Second, is one parent doing much more of the caregiving labor? That person is likely to see his or her income suffer over time. Third, how much do the parents share resources? Does that sharing make the situation fair? Will the sharing continue if the romantic relationship ends, especially if one of the parties gets a new romantic partner? Fourth, might it be best to memorialize in writing the parents' agreement about what is fair since attitudes can change over time?

Consider, for example, this *hypothetical situation*. Imagine one parent works part-time because of the child's needs or because both parents desire that arrangement. The other parent works full-time. After the workday concludes, both parents share the caregiving equally. For simplicity, assume that the full-time worker earns twice as much as the part-time worker.

Should the full-time worker turn over half of the income that he or she earned while the part-time worker fulfilled the full-time worker's caregiving responsibilities? Should the full-time worker pay the caregiving parent a salary? Should it be the amount that a day care provider or nanny would have received? Should the parents alternate by year the parent who works part-time? Should the full-time worker compensate the part-time worker with "in kind" benefits, such as the use of a car, free home repair, or on-demand babysitting? Should the full-time worker give the part-time worker money and time for a yearly vacation, especially if the part-time worker lost vacation benefits by going part-time? Should the full-time worker give the part-time worker a share of the full-time worker's future income after child support ends?

These questions suggest a range of possibilities. The parents themselves need to consider early on whether their arrangement is lopsided and how to make it fair.

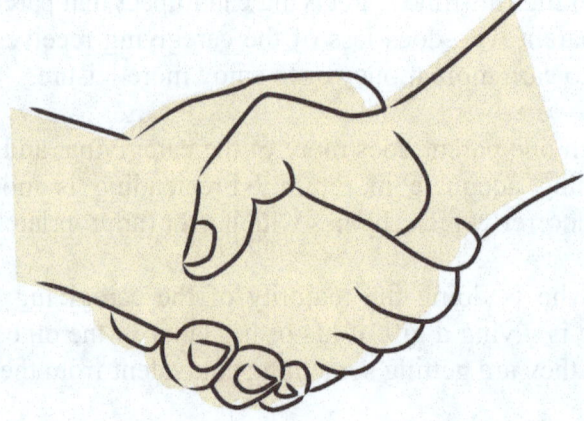

The bottom line is that a good parent-partner is not a schnorrer.

12) Remember that everything is bidirectional.

Yes, everything: both the good and the bad in a relationship go both ways. Great relationships do not involve one giver and one taker. They involve two givers, at least some of the time. In fact, once someone decides to be a giver, the other parent is much more likely to become a giver too. People tend to respond to kindness with kindness.

✔ **Fact:** Self-fulfilling prophecies exist.

If you treat your parent-partner like the parent-partner you want him or her to be, it is more likely that he or she will become the person you imagine.

The same is true in reverse. If you treat your parent-partner like he or she is an unsupportive person, then your parent-partner is more likely to become (or remain) unsupportive.

✔ **Fact:** "Gate closing" is a two-way phenomenon. After the romantic relationship ends, fathers sometimes criticize mothers for "closing the gate." They claim that mothers impose obstacles that make the fathers' relationships with their children difficult to maintain. Yet mothers who gate close typically describe unsupportive fathers. In fact, when fathers are supportive, mothers tend to be *gate openers* and go beyond what is legally required to keep the relationship between the father and child strong.

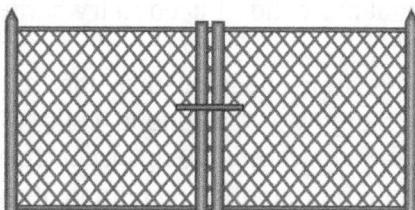

The same is true with *fighting*. Have you ever noticed how things can escalate when both parties are arguing? If one party says something hurtful, the other party tends to respond in a similar manner. Before you know it, things spiral downward. The relationship ends up, so to speak, in the toilet.

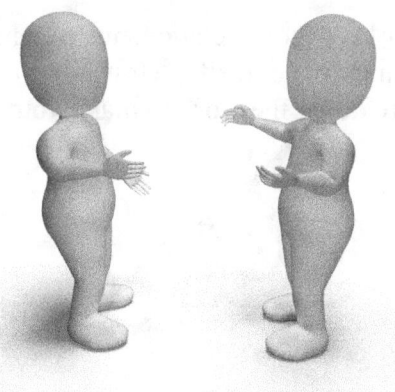

Here are some **tips**. When your partner says something critical about you, try to change the dynamics. Try not to respond by throwing out a criticism in response. It doesn't matter if you are right or wrong, good or bad at arguing, or too often the target of your partner's jibes.

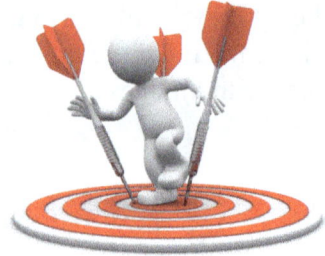

Instead, respond using one of these techniques.

Try, "I appreciate your feedback." Then change the subject.

Or try responding with an I-statement: "When you point out my flaws in the heat of an argument, it hurts my feelings. I want to address your concerns, but can we discuss them later, over dinner, when we are not fighting?" Recall that you can use a "child-statement" instead.

Or, if there might be merit in the criticism, show your partner that you've heard the concern and that you will work on a solution. For example, if he or she says, "It pisses me off that you don't return my phone calls," you could answer, "It makes you mad when I don't return your calls. You call me because you care about our child. I need to try harder to return your calls."

The conversation can obviously be more detailed than that example. The party who did not return the calls might want to share why the phone calls weren't answered (there was an emergency), or what would make answering them easier (perhaps if there were fewer), or whether an alternative method could be found for communicating (like texting), or whether there might be a bigger issue going on that should be addressed. For example, perhaps the caller is insecure about the status of the parties' romantic relationship, and the caller may need some reassurance or honest conversation.

The point is that relationships are bidirectional and *both* parties must respectfully communicate with each other, and work to keep the relationship on an upward trajectory.

After you've done something to keep your relationship moving in the right direction, reward yourself. At a minimum, murmur to yourself: "Upwards and onwards! To a great parent-partnership and beyond!" You are doing the work to make your romantic relationship last!

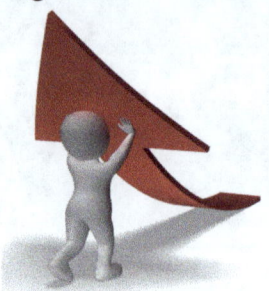

13) Have expectations about how parent-partners should act and apply those expectations to yourself and to your family and friends.

✔ **Fact:** Society's expectations can have a tremendous effect on how people act, feel, and see themselves. For example, library patrons are quiet in libraries because society expects people to be quiet. In contrast, people know that they can hoot and holler at a football game.

If family, friends, employers, and others treat you and your partner as "parent-partners," then you two will feel more like parent-partners and act accordingly. Similarly, if you treat others like parent-partners, then they are more likely to see themselves in that way too. Your expectations for other parent-partners will also reinforce the expectations that you have for your own parent-partnership.

✔ **Tip:** Start calling yourself a "parent-partner." Instead of introducing your child's other parent as your spouse, boyfriend, former spouse, or cohabitant, use the term "parent-partner." Ask others to refer to you both by that term.

✔ **Tip:** Start calling other parents who have a child in common "parent-partners." If people look puzzled, explain what the term means. It is not difficult to say, "The term means that the two people have a child in common and are committed to having a supportive relationship. Parent-partners exhibit fondness, flexibility, acceptance, togetherness, and empathy toward each other."

✔ **Tip:** Don't undermine other people's parent-partnerships. Couples are strengthened, and their relationships are made more enduring, if the relationship receives approval from others. Don't talk negatively about someone's parent-partner (unless an issue of safety is involved), and don't encourage a parent-partner to disrespect his or her parent-partner. Instead, reinforce the couple's shared commitment, created out of parenthood.

Everyone should expect parents with a child in common to be close friends and have an enduring supportive relationship, regardless of whether the couple is romantically involved, because good parent-partnerships benefit all of us. Economists estimate that family breakup and nonmarital childbearing costs society between $42 billion and $112 billion each year in program expenditures and reduced tax revenue. Those figures exclude the time courts spend resolving disputes between uncooperative parents. Its simply cheaper and better to help couples build strong relationships than to incur the costs of not having couples act as parent-partners. Public costs should decrease if people become more deliberate about their reproductive partners, work to keep their romantic relationships strong, and cooperate and support each other after their romantic relationships end and they repartner.

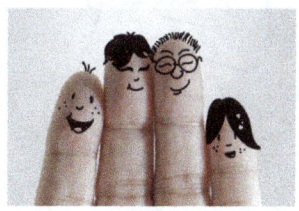

14) Being a successful parent-partner does not require a parent to stay in an unsafe situation.

Good parent-partners do not abuse the other parent. Period. "Abuse" here means both physical abuse and psychological abuse.

If you are the victim of abuse, you have every right to be safe. Abusive relationships are not supportive relationships. You can leave your abuser and still be a good parent-partner.

✔ **Fact**: Domestic violence harms the adult victim, but it can also harm the children. Children can suffer in various ways. Some kids get injured trying to protect their parents. Some kids become the batterer's targets. Some children suffer severe emotional problems well into adulthood because of their exposure to the violence. In one recent survey, 50% of the children exposed to domestic violence said that the violence was their most frightening experience ever. Moreover, children are disadvantaged when a parent is coping with the effects of domestic violence and therefore cannot parent to the best of his or her ability.

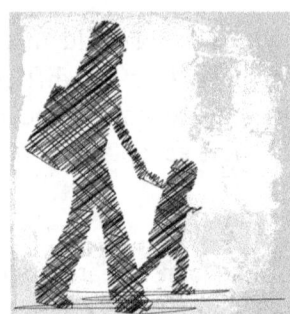

✔ **Fact:** You are more likely to be a victim of domestic violence if you have children. Parents are three times more likely to experience domestic violence than non-parents.

✔ **Fact:** Domestic violence often occurs during pregnancy. Domestic violence can start or escalate during pregnancy. A domestic violence victim faces three times the risk of homicide by her intimate partner once she becomes pregnant. The fetus can be harmed too. Domestic violence can cause miscarriage, preterm labor, fetal injury, and fetal death.

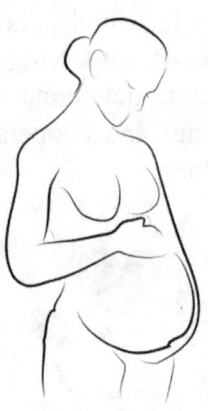

✔**Fact:** Psychological abuse is abuse. Psychological abuse can involve verbal or non-verbal behavior, such as constantly following the victim, invading the victim's personal space, stopping the victim from going somewhere, destroying the victim's possessions, controlling the victim's financial resources, and calling the victim degrading and insulting names. Psychological abuse can be more devastating to a victim than physical abuse. Psychological abuse can have both physical and/or mental repercussions. Psychological abuse can undermine the victim's parenting by signaling to the child that the parent is not worthy of respect.

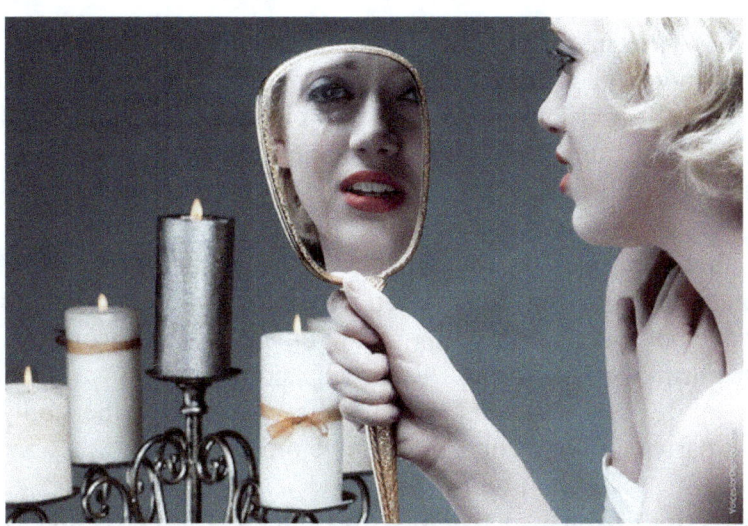

✔**Fact:** Not all abuse is the same. There is a difference between throwing a dish at someone's feet once in a long relationship and engaging in an ongoing campaign of terror. Similarly, not all psychologically aggressive acts are the same. There is a difference between using an insulting phrase and slashing someone's favorite dress with a knife. What makes some acts more problematic than others is the *context*; that is, the seriousness of the abuse depends on the nature of the acts, the actor's intent, and the effect on the victim. While physical and psychological abuse are *never* okay, abusive behavior is especially dangerous when it is part of a perpetrator's effort to dominate the victim, through pain, coercion, intimidation, and controlling tactics.

✔**Tip for the Victim**: If you have been injured or you are in danger of injury, call the police (911). You should also seek professional help immediately, in order to figure out how to stay safe, what to do next, and how to address the abuser's behavior. Stopping domestic violence can be difficult on your own, especially since leaving your abuser is one of the most dangerous times for victims, and your abuser may use your children as a way to keep you in the relationship. The National Domestic Violence Hotline can be reached at 1-800-799-7233 (TTY 1-800-787-3224). Your local domestic violence agency is also a good place to start. A local shelter can be found through this Web site, www.domesticshelters.org/, or by calling the National Domestic Violence Hotline.

✔**Tip for the Abuser:** If you are abusive toward your partner, stop it. Abusive behavior is wrong, often illegal, and hurts both your parent-partner and children.

35

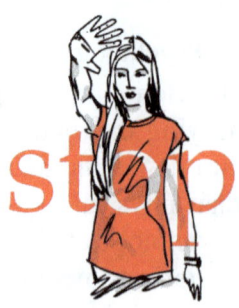

Resources exist to help you change your behavior. The National Domestic Violence Hotline is a good place to start. Among other things, the counselors there can talk to you about whether your behavior is abusive, its effect on others, and ways to change. The counselors can refer you to a batterer intervention program too. The phone number is 1−800−799−7233 (TTY 1−800−787−3224).

Until you get help (and you must do so immediately), you should consider using "time out to work out" as a strategy to avoid violence. When you feel a violent episode coming on, leave the area. Go away for one hour. Tell your partner that you are going to work out. During that hour, go work out. Don't drink or take drugs. Return if and when you can avoid violence. If the situation still feels toxic, wait until that toxicity disappears, and then only return to discuss matters when a third-party adult or a counselor can be present.

Is Obtaining a Protective Order Consistent with Being a Good Parent-Partner?

If you are a victim, you may be wondering, "How can I be a supportive parent-partner if I ask the court to keep my parent-partner away from me and our child." In fact, your abuser may ask you that question to stop you from accessing the legal remedies that you need.

Your safety and your children's safety must be your top priority. When your parent-partner abuses you, your parent-partner violates the most basic of the obligations of a parent-partnership. You are entitled to respond by accessing legal remedies.

Moreover, by keeping yourself and your children safe, you are not only being a good parent, but you are also being a good parent-partner. Think about this: When you stop your child from hurting another child, you are being a good parent because, among other things, you are trying to keep your child out of more trouble. Similarly, when you get a restraining order to stop your parent-partner from abusing you, you are trying to keep your parent-partner out of more trouble.

Most important, acting like a good parent-partner can be accomplished within the boundaries set by any court order. If a restraining order mandates that the other parent only have supervised visitation, "togetherness" might require overcoming this co-parenting challenge by transporting your child to the supervised visitation center, for example. Flexibility might require assuming more of the parenting burden while your parent-partner is prohibited from living with you. Acceptance might mean recognizing that your parent-partner is an abuser and unlikely to change.

Child abuse raises many of the same points for a parent-partnership as those just discussed. Child abuse is discussed below under point 16.

15) Consider creating some legal obligations to reflect and reinforce your commitment.

Two parents can decide to act like model parent-partners without memorializing their agreement in writing. Parents don't need to put their commitment into a legally binding document. Yet there may be certain advantages to creating some legally binding obligations. For example, crafting an agreement before conception can focus a couple on whether they are ready, willing, and able to commit to a parent-partnership. The formality of a contract conveys the seriousness of the step being taken. In addition, legally binding obligations — in the form of a contract — can keep people on track when their original goals fade over time.

Anyone who plans on entering a parent-partner contract should consult with a lawyer to ensure that the agreement is enforceable. Spouses, in particular, may find a court reluctant to enforce a parent-partner contract for a host of reasons. While a court might be more willing to enforce a contract between unmarried parents, a court still might not enforce the contract in certain circumstances, including if the court thinks that the parties contracted for sex. Contracting parties should also consult with lawyers to get advice on provisions to include in a contract. Lawyers also help parties avoid unanticipated consequences.

What obligations should go into a contract? There are endless subjects about which parent-partners might contract. Think about including provisions that would address big topics, endure over time, and reinforce the meaning of the parent-partner role. Consequently, don't detail who will take out the trash, wash the clothes, or pay for groceries. Too many details will become cumbersome and undermine the flexibility that parent-partners need. You wouldn't want to create provisions that would be hard to follow or that would become outdated quickly.

The following suggestions for contract provisions are loosely based on the recommendations offered in *A Parent-Partner Status for American Family Law*. That book suggests that the law should automatically impose the following obligations on all parents with a child in common. These legal obligations would help people recognize that they are parent-partners and how society expects parent-partners to act. Although the book predicts that very few people would ever contract for these legal obligations on their own (and therefore recommends that they be automatically imposed by law), nothing prohibits parent-partners from contracting to address these points or others like them. To be clear, these provisions might not be enforceable in court. But, then again, if the contract helped the parents have a solid parent-partnership, the provisions would never need to be enforced anyway.

The "Not-a-Contract" Contract. If entering a legally binding contract seems daunting, or if you would prefer not to obtain legal advice, consider entering an agreement that is not legally enforceable (perhaps using this form). Be sure to put at the top of the document that the agreement is *NOT* meant to be a legally binding contract. Rather, the "non-contract" would simply state your and your partner's intentions and expectations. Even without a legally enforceable document, the writing might convey the serious nature of the new relationship and set the right expectations.

SAMPLE PARENT-PARTNER AGREEMENT

Recitals

1) _____ and _____ are parents of _____, born _____.

2) _____ and _____[hereafter referred to as "the parent-partners"] consider themselves to be parent-partners and family.

3) Both parent-partners are committed to the following: to having a solid parenting-partnership regardless of what happens to their romantic relationship; to supporting each other in the parenting activity; and to acting kindly toward each other outside the parenting context.

4) The parent-partners are entering this agreement in order to reinforce their commitment to have a supportive, cooperative partnership.

As such, the parent-partners agree to the following:

1) *Duty to Aid.* We agree to help the other if the other is ever physically imperiled and it is reasonable to do so. For example, if one of us falls ill and needs an ambulance, and the other person is around and can call for an ambulance, that person will be obligated to do so.

2) *Duty Not to Abuse.* We agree never to abuse each other, either physically or psychologically.

3) *Duty to Undertake Relationship Work.* We agree to engage in educational programs or couples counseling during pregnancy or within three months after the birth of our child in order to keep our relationship strong. We also agree to seek counseling at the demise of our romantic relationship. We will explore the possibility of reconciliation, and if we do not reconcile we will work together to have a strong friendship.

4) *Duty to Treat Each Other With Loyalty When Contracting.* In the future, we may want to enter another formal agreement regarding our relationship. The agreement might be a pre-nuptial agreement, post-nuptial agreement, cohabitation agreement, agreement related to caregiver compensation, or an agreement to settle our affairs after we breakup. Regardless, we agree to treat each other honestly and fairly when we enter or enforce such a contract. Specifically, we agree to the following: not to exert undue pressure on the other party; to disclose sufficient information so that the other person's decision is informed; and not to enforce an agreement that becomes very unfair over time.

5) *Duty to Give Care or Share.* We agree to share equally our obligation to give physical care to our child, subject to a court order allocating custody in a different manner. If one of us does a disproportionate amount of the caregiving, we agree that such person should be compensated fairly for that effort. We agree to come to an agreement about a fair arrangement at the time disproportionate caregiving begins, and we will periodically reassess whether our arrangement is a fair one and adjust compensation accordingly. If we cannot agree on what is fair compensation, we agree to resolve our disagreement with the help of a mediator.

We intend these obligations to be legally binding until our child becomes 18 years old.

Nothing in this agreement is intended to waive or alter any legal remedy or protections that a party might otherwise have under the law.

_____   _____
Name   Date

_____   _____
Name   Date

Subscribed and sworn to before me, this _____[day of month] day of _____[month], 2015 by _____ and _____

[Notary Seal:]

State of _____, County of _____

_____
[signature of Notary]

_____
[typed name of Notary]

NOTARY PUBLIC

MY COMMISSION EXPIRES

16) Continue acting as parent-partners after the romantic relationship ends.

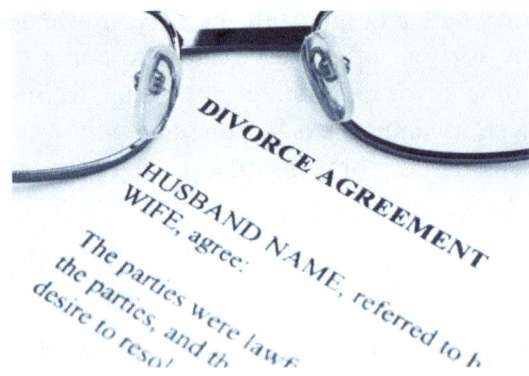

It happens. It may have already happened. It may happen in the future. "It," of course, is a breakup.

Although it may never happen, no romantic relationship is indestructible. After all, relationships between humans involve humans, and humans are not perfect. In fact, humans can sometimes be downright idiotic and irrational. Even if humans were perfect, however, humans' feelings and tastes change over time. As a result, romantic relationships can sour.

While the breakup of the parents' romantic relationship is often a big deal, the breakup does not terminate the parent-partnership. A parent-partnership is **not** a romantic relationship. It exists even after the romantic relationship ends. A parent-partnership is kind of like herpes in that way (yes, that analogy is icky, but you get the point).

Often bad feelings accompany a breakup. A parent may be sad, angry, resentful, or hurt. Consequently, that parent may withdraw, or that parent may share everything with everyone. Alternatively, a parent may be coping just fine. That parent may feel strong and capable, and even excited about his or her newfound freedom. Parents may have the same feelings when they split, or they may have the opposite feelings. One parent may be sad and the other parent may be happy. With all of these possibilities, it is no wonder that country music artists commonly sing about breakups.

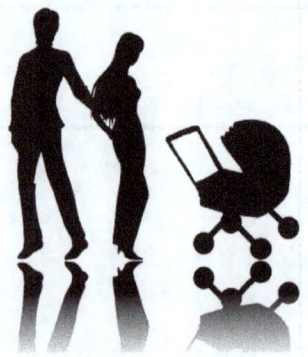

Turmoil is very common during the early years after a divorce or the breakup of an unmarried relationship. For some couples, it never ends.

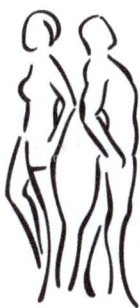

Parents must not allow their child to experience their hostility. A breakup is not the child's fault. The child should never be put in the middle of the adults' disagreements or be exposed to the parents' fighting or arguing. Never put down the other parent, blame the other parent, ask the child to take a side, or ask the child to keep secrets. Don't do these things regardless of whether the other parent is present or absent when you speak about him or her. Don't do these things no matter how much you dislike the other parent or believe your feelings are justified.

Remember, your child has half of the other parent's genetic material. *When you put down the other parent, you are putting down your child.*

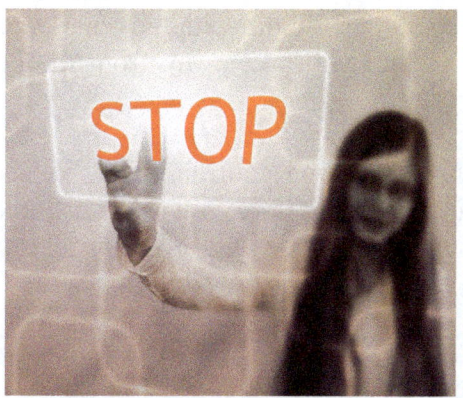

Some couples can successfully navigate a breakup on their own, but many cannot. **Professionals** are very helpful for two reasons.

First, professionals can help you and your partner explore whether ending the romantic relationship is really the best outcome for your child. Sometimes people want to split up because they feel they "have grown apart," or they feel their partner "is not affectionate," or they "don't feel the same passion." A counselor can often successfully address these problems with the parties, or at least help parties consider whether these reasons justify a breakup. Consequently, parents should try counseling. After all, children do better when their parents remain in a romantic relationship (as long as the parents do not have a high-conflict relationship).

Sometimes one parent must address a personal problem, such as mental illness or addiction, before reconciliation can occur. The National Alliance on Mental Illness, 1-800-950-6264, Alcoholics Anonymous, www.aa.org/, and Narcotics Anonymous, www.na.org/, are all helpful places to start.

If one or both parents are unwilling to stay in the romantic relationship, perhaps because change and forgiveness are not in the cards, or because the relationship cannot be rebuilt into a healthy relationship, then life must still go on. People end their romantic relationships every day, and the adults survive the experience. That explains why we have great songs like "Survivor" by Destiny's Child and "I Will Survive" by Gloria Gaynor.

The second reason to see a professional at the end of the romantic relationship is because a professional can help parents minimize the harm that their child may experience from the breakup by maximizing the chances that the parents will be friends after their romantic relationship ends. As one leader in the field said, a professional can help parents close the door softly instead of with a thud. A professional can also help parents keep the door open when that is best for their child.

When the relationship ends, and the parties are unwinding their emotional connection, parents have to *address their children's needs*. Children require a lot of love and attention at this point. Each parent must nurture his or her relationship with the child. Children need information and comfort, as well as reassurance about receiving each parent's current and future love. Among other things, you should listen to your child and assure your child that you and the other parent are parent-partners and that you will continue to have a supportive friendship. Kids want and need to hear that message. Kids want security. Kids need to know that you care enough about them that you will keep your parent-partnership with the other person strong. If you do keep your parent-partnership strong, your child will take away from the breakup a life lesson about the importance of responsibility.

There are many good books about meeting your children's needs during a breakup or divorce. Look at these types of resources long before you ever get into court. While a court may eventually order you and your partner into a co-parenting class that addresses some of these matters, your child needs you to be a responsible parent from the first moment that you and your partner decide to call it quits.

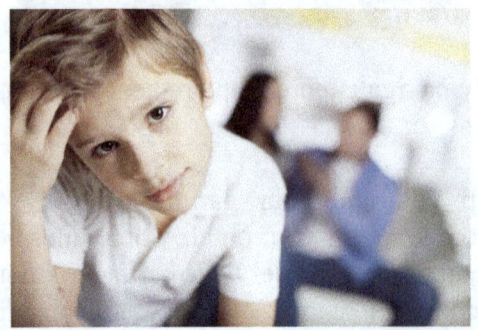

After the romantic relationship ends, being a supportive parent-partner is not always easy. Nonetheless, you should strive for this outcome because it is what is best for your child. If you have followed the parent-partner philosophy from the beginning of your relationship, you will have a much easier time at breakup than someone who hears about the philosophy for the first time at the end of his or her romantic relationship. Nevertheless, you may never have imagined that your romantic relationship would end at all, so there will still be new challenges when it does even if you and your parent-partner have had a strong parent-partnership all along.

The main challenge will be working together to minimize the breakup's effect on your child. Questions to consider include the following: How can we work together to keep both parents *actively involved* in our child's life? How can we minimize the disruption that living in two homes might otherwise cause our child? How can we reduce the economic effects of family breakup for our child? How can we ensure our child's life opportunities are not diminished because of our breakup? How can we minimize our expenses by acting as a team? How can we share resources? What contributions of food, diapers, college tuition, etc. can we each make to benefit our child, in addition to our legally required contributions? How can we cooperate so that both parents can advance professionally in ways that will benefit our child one day; can we help each other attend college or have time for homework?

Warning! Child support is *not* high enough to eliminate the economic effects of a family breakup. Additional cooperation is critical.

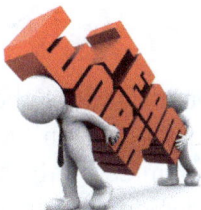

There are four items that can make a *huge* difference to your child's experience during and after your breakup: parenting plans; co-parenting styles; mediation; and gate opening. Please consider the following.

Parenting Plans

Many states require parents to have a parenting plan when they use the courts to divorce, or to obtain a custody or paternity order. A parenting plan lays out how parents can co-parent together after the end of their romantic relationship. The plan addresses issues like the child's schedule, who makes which decisions about the child's life (for example, religion, education, etc.), how the parents will communicate, and how parents will resolve differences regarding child-related issues. The parenting plan helps the parents work as a team after they split up. It provides parents with a guide in case the parents' informal arrangements break down. As Benjamin Franklin apparently once said, "If you fail to plan, you are planning to fail."

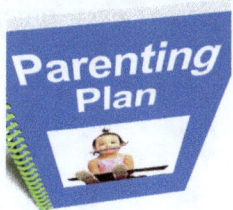

If the parents cannot agree to a parenting plan, many courts will create one. However, the outcome will be much better if the parents can design their own plan. No one knows a child and the child's needs as well as the parents. The plan is the beginning of the teamwork that is essential to successful co-parenting after a breakup. The Web has many examples of parenting plans; search for "parenting plan template" or "parenting plan sample." Some states, like Oregon, put a court-created form online. Court Web sites are a useful place to start looking when you are trying to find a model.

It often is very useful to have someone assist you and your partner with this plan. The third party can keep you both focused on the task at hand, suggest topics that should be addressed in the plan, and help resolve some disagreements. Therefore, consider asking an attorney, custody evaluator, parenting coordinator, social worker, mediator, or a psychologist to help you draft the plan. If the disagreements are too great to be resolved over the kitchen table or in a professional's office, mediation can be very helpful (see below).

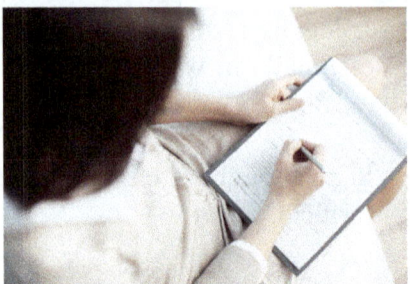

As you create the parenting plan, remember that it is about your *child's* needs. Also, remember to keep your child out of the fray as you draft it. Don't ask your child to decide with whom he or she wants to live. Listen if your child volunteers information, but you and your partner (as the parents) or the judge (as the judge) must decide what is best for your child.

Methods of Co-Parenting

There are three styles of co-parenting after parents part ways: conflicted, disengaged, or supportive. Which do you think is the best for children? Here is a hint: the options are arranged from worst to best.

Conflicted co-parenting is **never** good for kids. Even if this is your co-parenting style, do not put down the other parent or exhibit conflict in front of your child.

Disengaged or "parallel parenting" has become the most common form of co-parenting following a breakup. Parents with this style typically raise their child along separate tracks. While there are different degrees of parallel parenting, some parents hardly interact at all and restrict communication to written correspondence about child-related subjects. Typically, parents who use parallel parenting do not see each other in person. It is a very business-like arrangement.

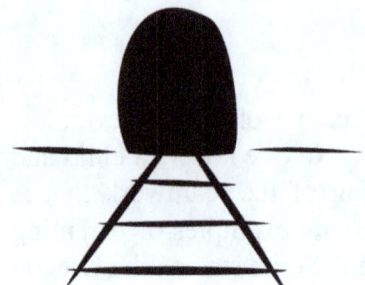 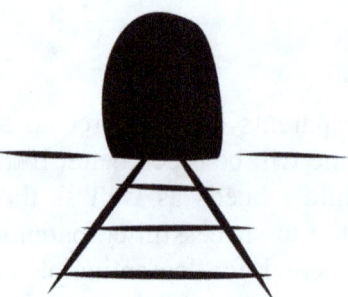

Although many parents use this technique, its popularity is not a good reason to select parallel parenting. To coin an old adage, "Just because all of the other lemmings are jumping off of the cliff doesn't mean that you should jump too." Parent-partners should seriously question whether "parallel parenting" is best for their children. While parallel parenting is a *great* approach for couples that have high-conflict relationships, this arrangement can cause children to miss certain benefits if their parents could instead have a supportive co-parenting relationship.

A supportive co-parenting relationship means that both parents will act as a team, exhibiting fondness, acceptance, togetherness, empathy, and flexibility to the greatest degree possible. Big decisions will be made together, there will be gate opening (see below for the meaning of this term), and there will not be conflict (or it will be successfully suppressed).

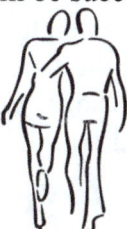

Supportive co-parenting has obvious benefits for the parents. Imagine sharing exciting news about your child with the other parent. Imagine the other parent sharing exciting news about your child with you. Imagine attending parent-teacher conferences together. Imagine one day attending graduations and weddings together, and being proud of what you both have accomplished by raising your child together. Imagine going on a family vacation together and having a good time.

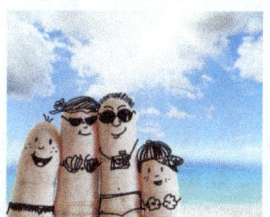

Wait a minute! Of course, the ability to vacation together is not actually a requirement for a cooperative and successful partnership. Many couples that co-parent supportively never vacation together. Even best friends may not want to vacation together! Everyone has a limit! While a trip to Alaska with your children may make its tourism slogan accurate, *"Beyond Your Dreams, Within Your Reach,"* traveling with your ex-spouse too may turn that slogan into, *"Beyond Your Comfort Level."* The point is that you don't need to vacation together so long as you generally have a cooperative and supportive co-parenting arrangement.

Supportive co-parenting does not mean the parents are entitled to venture into past relationship issues or burden the other parent with excessive communication. While it is appropriate to call the other parent and ask, "Can you take Jane to ballet class this Wednesday because I have to work," it is inappropriate to call the other parent and ask, "Can we talk about why you fooled around with that hideous person you met on Tinder?"

Supportive co-parents, like good friends, try not to push buttons or respond negatively when buttons are pushed. Good friends take things in stride, realizing that the relationship itself is more important than "winning" an argument. Good friends listen to each other. Good friends want others (here, their children) to know that they are good friends and care about each other.

Relationships change over time and you and your partner can move from supportive parenting to parallel parenting or from parallel parenting to supportive parenting. However, there is a risk if you start with parallel parenting, you may never switch to supportive parenting. People become set in their ways. In fact, there is a real risk that one parent may disengage during parallel parenting and may even become an absent parent. If you have the ability, start by trying supportive co-parenting. It may not be as easy as parallel parenting, but who ever said that parenting, or co-parenting, was easy? Ask professionals to help you and your partner try it.

Regardless of the approach, recognize that you cannot control your parent-partner's parenting. Nor should you want to do so unless your parent-partner is endangering your child, in which case you must. That is not to say that you cannot respectfully raise your concerns (using the "I-statement"), but you must chose your battles carefully so not to cause a conflicted co-parenting arrangement. Ultimately, you must accept the other parent's parenting decisions if there is no danger. By accepting the other parent's decisions, you are accepting the other person as a parent. This acceptance then conveys to your child that he or she has your permission to love both of you unconditionally.

Regardless of your co-parenting approach, there are many "skills" that can be helpful to successful co-parenting, including how to communicate in a way that decreases the potential for conflict. This book is not about those skills, but you can find such resources on-line. One free and excellent resource is the "Co-parenting Communication Guide" written by the Arizona chapter of the Association of Family and Conciliation Courts. You can find it here: www.afccnet.org/Portals/0/PDF/AzAFCC%20Coparenting%20Communication%20Guide.pdf

Mediation

Research shows that parents who use mediation instead of adjudication to resolve their custody disputes are much more likely to have both parents actively involved in their children's lives over a decade later. Mediation sets the tone for working together over time. Mediation also helps spare children the negative outcomes that can occur when the parents are hostile and in court fighting over custody.

Experienced mediators have a variety of techniques that can help you and your partner focus on the future and reach an agreement. Some programs even include the child in the mediation session, but that is typically done just to ensure that his or her needs are being met.

You should investigate the mediation option. Mediation may not be appropriate, however, if there is domestic violence in your relationship. A good mediator will explore with you the appropriateness of mediation before you engage in it.

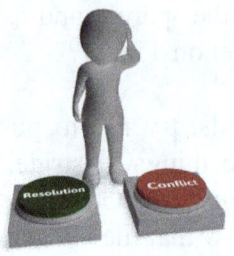

Gate Opening

Regardless of whether the child lives primarily with one parent after breakup or evenly with both parents, schedules can sometimes become difficult, unworkable, or disadvantageous.

For example, imagine the child spends Mondays with one parent, but the other parent's office is having a "take your daughter to work day" on a particular Monday. The other parent wants to involve his daughter in this event, but cannot do so without a schedule change. When such an accommodation is made, it is called "gate opening." These accommodations are not legally required, but they benefit the child and reflect supportive, cooperative parenting.

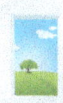

Another example: Imagine one parent is throwing a party to celebrate the fact that his son made the honor roll. The other parent would love to attend the party, but she is not legally entitled to do so. If the party thrower opened the gate to the other parent by inviting her to the party, both parents could participate in the event to celebrate their son's achievement. The son would appreciate that outcome.

Parents should strive to be gate openers. In certain situations, gate opening is especially important. For example, when parents live far apart, the custodial parent should encourage a child to call the other parent, write letters to the other parent, and visit the other parent. The custodial parent has considerable control over the future of the child's relationship with the other parent.

Warning! Much of the above information does not apply if there has been child abuse or neglect by a parent. In such a situation, the protective parent should contact an attorney or professional for help. That National Child Abuse Hotline can be reached at 1-800-4-A-CHILD (1-800-422-4453). Depending upon the issues, the court may take a number of actions, including requiring the abusive or neglectful parent to attend parenting classes, to submit to drug or alcohol treatment, and to see the child only in a supervised setting. In some cases, although rarely, the court may preclude all contact between the child and the abusive or neglectful parent.

Warning! If there has been domestic violence between the parties, much of the above information does not apply. Domestic violence harms children in many ways (see point 14 above). In such a situation, the target of the abuse should contact an attorney or other professional for guidance.

Custody Orders. This section has not focused on the parents' formal child custody arrangement after breakup. Why? The legal arrangement is actually a lot less important than having a supportive partnership. Parents with a supportive partnership will generally prefer joint legal and physical custody, but they will act as if they have that arrangement regardless of what the custody order actually says. In fact, there may be financial or other reasons for a different arrangement. Talk to a lawyer about the options.

17) Continue to act like parent-partners through repartnering.

Repartnering is a fact of life. Divorced parents often remarry or cohabit with new partners. Unmarried parents also frequently move on to other partners, either marrying them or cohabiting with them. It is not unusual for people to become parents with their new partners. Nor is it unusual for these subsequent relationships to end one day.

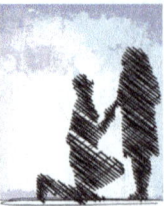

When one parent enters a romantic relationship with someone else, it can be challenging for the other parent. Repartnering can strain a couple's co-parenting relationship and cause the child stress. Some parents feel pushed to the side by the new stepparent or romantic partner. If both parents have children with others, they can be pulled in opposite directions. Parallel parenting tends to become more common after repartnering.

Good parent-partners have strong parent-partnerships even after one or both parents repartner.

✔ **Tip: Remember f.f.a.t.e**: fondness, flexibility, acceptance, togetherness, and empathy. These traits are really important to exhibit as repartnering occurs.

For the repartnering parent, *empathy* and *acceptance* mean *going slowly* to establish new relationships because repartnering can be hard for the other parent and the child. It also means considering your parent-partner's feelings as you repartner. For example, tell your parent-partner when you are going to introduce your new partner to the child and solicit input on how the child should address your new partner.

For the non-repartnering parent, *acceptance* means acknowledging that your parent-partner probably will repartner. Support the repartnered parent's happiness to the best of your abilities. After all, he or she is still the parent of your child. In addition, you will want the same courtesy when you repartner one day.

Togetherness requires that both parent-partners work jointly to overcome this co-parenting challenge. The parents must listen respectfully to each other's concerns and show *flexibility* in addressing them. Concerns that relate to the children's safety must be taken seriously.

Parent-partners must ensure that their new partners have the *maturity* not to undermine the parent-partnership. New partners must recognize that parent-partners will remain important family members to each other despite the repartnering. New partners should applaud the couple's co-parenting commitment, and must accept the ongoing effort that their commitment will require. New partners must not undermine the parent-partnership. When the new partner shows support for the parent-partnership, both parent-partners should in turn show appreciation to the new partner. A love-fest is not required, just good ole respect and gratitude. Saying thank you, for example, would be appropriate (a gift certificate to a coffee shop wouldn't hurt either)!

18) Spread the Word

As you now know, the parent-partner relationship is an important one that deserves the attention of parents themselves, but also of society. You can help the parent-partner concept become socially significant by spreading the word.

There are at least two ways to spread the word about the parent-partner concept. One is simply by living your life as a good parent-partner. This will prompt some questions from others about the concept (for example, others may ask you about the term "parent-partner"). Living your life as a parent-partners will also spread the concept because you will make it much more likely that your children, and their children, will be good parent-partners one day too. Children learn by watching you and your parent-partner treat each other well. When your children grow up and become parents themselves, your children will be much more likely to seek a partner who can commit to a solid parent-partnership. Like the pebble that is thrown into the pond, your actions will have a ripple effect.

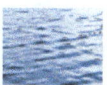

The other way to spread the word is by actually spreading the word. Here are some **tips** for how to get the message out.

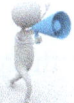

✔Recommend that friends and family learn about the parent-partner concept.

✔Add a link to the www.parent-partners.com Web site at the end of your emails or texts and suggest that people check it out.

✔Send this book to your children's health teacher and suggest that the teacher incorporate this concept into the school curriculum.

✔Write a letter to the editor of your local paper and suggest that people consider the possibilities presented by the parent-partner concept.

✔Send a copy of this book to a lawmaker. Ask for laws that would create a parent-partner status.

✔Buy a parent-partner tattoo on the www.parent-partners.com Web site and wear it proudly (yes, such an item exists). There you will also find "child of parent-partners" bibs, "parent-partner" t-shirts, "child of parent-partner" t-shirts, and other parent-partner gear.

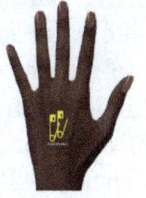 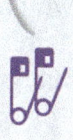

19) Ask your library to order the academic book, *A Parent-Partner Status for American Family Law,* **and take a look at it.**

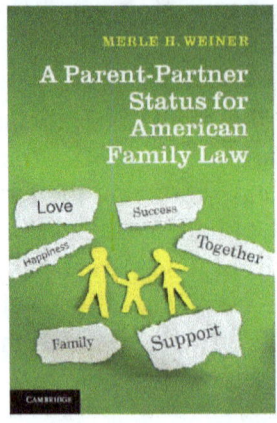

Now that you've considered the parent-partner concept, you may be interested in learning more about the need for the legal status, the research behind the proposal, and the details of the proposed parent-partner status. If so, please consider reading *A Parent-Partner Status for American Family Law.*

A Parent-Partner Status for American Family Law argues that society should make the birth or adoption of a child a significant event for the parents' legal relationship to each other. It suggests that society should create a legal status that would automatically apply to parents who have a child in common. Five core legal obligations would constitute the status and obligate the parents to each other in various ways. These legal obligations would also create and shape the social role of parent-partner. Lawmakers would have to decide which core legal obligations should be imposed on parent-partners, but the book recommends the legal obligations that were suggested for the contract that was discussed in point 15 earlier. Any legal obligations chosen should reflect those norms that make people successful parent-partners: flexibility, fondness, acceptance, togetherness, and empathy. The legal obligations would last until the parents' child turned eighteen years old, although the social role of "parent-partner" would continue throughout the parents' lives. None of the legal obligations would obligate the government or third parties to provide anything to parent-partners. Nor would the status obligate parent-partners to do anything for the government or third parties. Any legal obligations would arise only between the parents themselves, and only for couples that had a child after the proposed status became law.

Such a status would have many advantages. People would become more deliberate about when and with whom they have a child. After all, parenthood would create legal obligations between the parents for the next 18 years. There would be clear social norms about the nature of the parent-partner relationship: it should be a supportive partnership. Because there would be a social role, people who occupied it would be likely to act in accordance with the societal expectations. The status would be a fairer way to structure the law. Right now, nonmarital children have no legal structure at all that guides their parents' relationship in the direction of a strong partnership. The same is true for children of divorced parents. The status might also foster love between the parents and promote civic virtue. All of these possibilities are explained in detail in the academic book. The possible disadvantages are also addressed there.

Why Do We Need A Parent-Partner Legal Status?

You may be saying to yourself, "I just read this entire book and you told me how to be a parent-partner without any legal change at all. Why does society need legal change?" There are two reasons.

First, not everyone will decide to become a parent-partner. Unfortunately, not every couple that has children or that will have children will read this book, hear about the idea, or decide to commit to a parent-partnership. That is why the parent-partner status and role should arise automatically. Then becoming a "parent-partner" would be just like becoming a "parent." As soon as a biological connection between a parent and child were established, the social role and legal status would kick in to govern the parents' relationship.

Otherwise, if people can elect whether to become a parent-partner, then one parent may refuse to do so. This can leave the other parent without a legal remedy for unfair and harmful behavior. It can also leave children without a legal structure to guide their parents' relationships. It also means that the law would not deter unprotected sexual intercourse by those who don't want a parent-partnership, and those people are the very individuals who need to be deterred.

Second, an automatic legal status is the surest way to create a new social role. The law sends a very strong message when it creates a mandatory status. People would take notice of a new status. Such a response is important, not only for making the law effective, but also for creating a new social role.

A social role? If you are a "mother" or a "father," you have a social role. "Spouse" is a social role too. Social roles affect people's behavior even more than the law itself. Just think about the social role of "spouse." A "spouse" is not supposed to cheat. Others convey that message all the time. The friend who says, "Hey, don't flirt, you are married," the magazine article that tells engaged couples to throw away their "little black books," and the wedding band, all convey and reinforce social expectations. Sure, there are competing messages, like from the Web site Ashley Madison (with its slogan, "Life is short. Have an affair."). Those competing messages perhaps explain why 25 percent of married men and 15 percent of married women do cheat. Yet there is a lot less cheating overall because of the general social expectations associated with the role of spouse. *We need to create a social role for people who have a child in common. That social role would come with social expectations about the parents' relationship to each other.*

As you now know, *a parent-partner is not the same thing as a "mom" or "dad."* The term "mom" or "dad" describes the relationship of a parent to a child. When a child is born or adopted, the "mom" and "dad" (or, in some instances, mom and mom or dad and dad) have that role automatically.

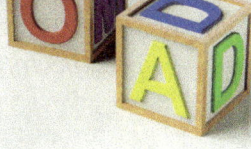

We have *social expectations* for how parents should act toward their child and feel about their child. These social expectations exist as soon as the child is born. We would probably agree that society expects good parents to love their child, to care for their child, to support their child to the best of their abilities (both emotionally and materially), and to nurture their child to become a responsible, productive adult.

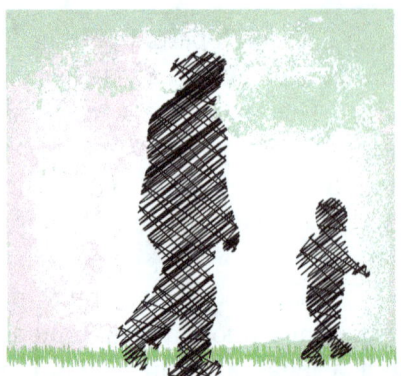

Laws that set a minimum level of acceptable parental behavior shape society's expectations. Consider the many laws that govern the parent-child relationship. For example, parents must not neglect or abuse their children; otherwise, the government may intervene for the child's protection. Similarly, the law requires parents to support their children financially and to send their children to school. While the government may have passed some of these laws to reflect existing societal expectations about parental behavior, the laws also reinforce those societal expectations. The laws help us understand, for example, that parents must educate their children. Most parents, of course, comply with the law voluntarily by sending their children to school. Yet the law has shaped our own understanding of what it means to be a good parent and also fosters compliance. Laws that prohibit employers from discriminating against women in the job market similarly shape our ideas about whose job it is to change diapers at home. The parent-partner status would work similarly. As one legal scholar noted, family law has a wide reach and low-intensity. It sets the boundaries of acceptable conduct. It guides most people's behavior without the law ever being invoked directly in a court of law by the parties affected.

Contrast the societal expectations for the parent-child relationship with the absence of societal expectations for the relationship between parents of the same child. Can you describe society's expectations for the parents' relationship to each other? This book just argued that we *should* expect parents to have a supportive, cooperative partnership from the get-go, and to exhibit the qualities captured by the acronym f.f.a.t.e., but do we? Do we have any expectations for how unmarried parents should treat each other? Even for married parents, do we have any laws that convey an expectation that the parents stay together if that is best for their child, or at least act like a supportive team (not just a cooperative team) if the parents divorce? We certainly do not prohibit divorce for such couples with children or require that the parents consider reconciliation. The law does encourage parents to support the child's relationship with the other parent after breakup, but the law doesn't encourage the parents to support *each other*. In fact, most married and unmarried couples cannot name any changes to their own legal relationship that arose from having a baby. *As a consequence, the social expectations for two parents who have a child in common are virtually nonexistent.*

Consider what the absence of legal obligations signals. For example, the law imposes no obligation on a divorced or unmarried parent to call 911 when the other parent is injured and dying in the street, although it imposes that obligation on spouses. The absence of a legal obligation for all parents is quite sickening, and not only because the child would suffer from the death of the injured parent. Rather, society should expect better of two people who have a child in common and should afford the injured parent a remedy when the other parent fails to act appropriately. When the law doesn't afford a remedy, it suggests that a parent need not assist the one who is injured.

What do we call the relationship between two people who have a child in common? There is **no** term.

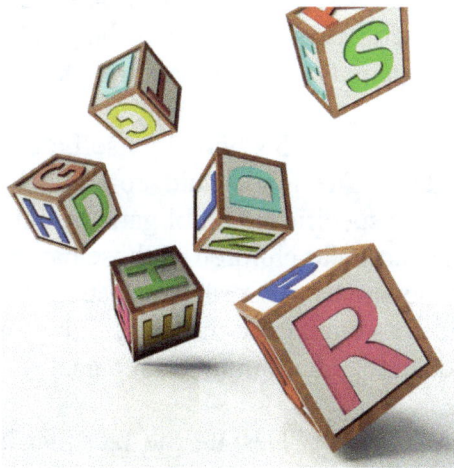

Unlike the term mom or dad, *we don't even have a name to describe the relationship between the two individuals who have a child together*. We can't call two individuals who have a child together "spouses" because unmarried couples have babies and because married people frequently divorce and are no longer spouses. We don't have different terms for married couples with and without children, even though a child changes the everyday interaction between married parties in fundamental ways. Terms like "baby mama" are unhelpful because they are often used as a put-down and such phrases cast the parents' relationship to each other only as an indirect one, that is, as a relationship that only exists through the child. It does not suggest a direct family relationship between the parents themselves. "Co-parents" does not work either because that term usually refers to people who are parenting together after the end of their romantic relationship. However, most couples start parenting together during a romantic relationship. Co-parent also only refers to that aspect of the couple's relationship that deals with co-parenting, but that behavior is subsumed within a broader relationship that is important to keep friendly and to characterize as a family relationship. *Isn't it odd that U.S. society has no term that describes the relationship of parents with a child in common?*

We need a name for that relationship and we need social expectations for it too! If a cooperative and supportive relationship between parents is best for children, then society should convey those expectations. Society should have *some laws* that govern the parents' relationship to each other to help create and reflect the necessary social expectations. If society imposed some legal obligations that set a minimum level of socially acceptable behavior between parents with a child in common, society would be on its way to creating the *social role of "parent-partner."*

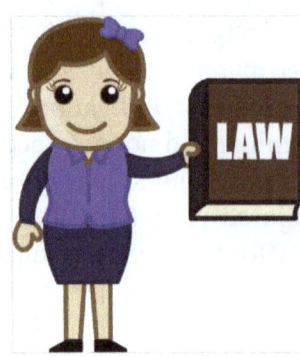

As mentioned, *A Parent-Partner Status for American Family Law* argues that the law should impose an automatic "parent-partner" status on parents who have a child in common. The status would impose a legal structure on parents and help create a social role.

While such a status might not be needed if this book by itself created a social role, more than this book will undoubtedly be needed. The law would be a much more effective way to affect widespread social change. Plus, the specific legal obligations that constituted the status would be beneficial to the parents, and the particular children of those parents, who needed to invoke them. For example, if a parent could obtain a court order to restrain the other parent's psychological abuse, the abused parent would be advantaged and the children would be too. In addition, the availability of the order might deter the abuse in the first place!

Here is a brief description of the book: "Despite the fact that becoming a parent is a pivotal event, the birth or adoption of a child has little significance for parents' legal relationship to each other. Instead, the law relies upon marriage, domestic partnerships, contracts, and some equitable remedies to set the parameters of the legal obligations between the parents. With high rates of nonmarital childbirth and divorce, the current approach to regulating the legal relationship of parents is outdated. A new legal and social structure is needed to encourage parents to act as supportive partners and to deter uncommitted couples from having children. This book is the first of its kind to propose a new 'parent-partner' status for American family law. This book includes a detailed discussion of the benefits of the status, as well as specific recommendations for legal obligations."

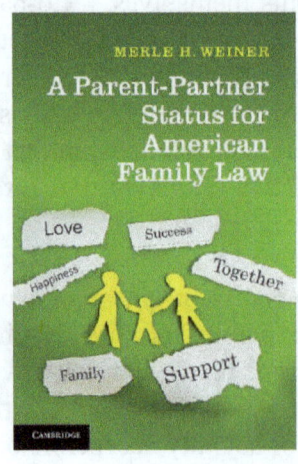

Here is the Table of Contents:

1) The disconnect between the facts and the law
2) The absence of a parent-partner status
3) The inadequacy of existing constructs
4) Reform efforts: slowly moving forward
5) The new status in theoretical perspective
6) The benefits of the new status for children
7) The benefits of the new status for the community
8) Ambitions for the new status
9) New nonmonetary obligations
10) A new relationship work obligation
11) New obligations with financial implications
12) Possible concerns about the parent-partner status

A Parent-Partner Status for American Family Law can be purchased at
www.cambridge.org/9781107088085

✔ **Tip:** The book is not cheap. Ask your local library to purchase it and then borrow it for free.

> The idea behind the parent-partner status is the following: An automatic parent-partner status would help create the role of "parent-partner" in society, provide a framework for the type of relationship parents should have with each other, help people consider before conception whether they are willing and capable of being in a parent-partnership with the other person, and guide peoples' actions in ways that are beneficial for their children.

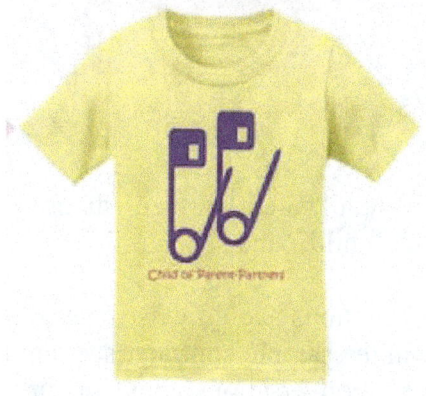

20) Ask your state representative to create a status that would apply to all parent-partners.

A legal status makes sense because parents who have a child in common *should* act like parent-partners. But we do so little as a society to encourage that behavior. It is simply too little, too late to have co-parenting classes at the time parents go to court to resolve a custody dispute. It harms children when society is so indifferent to whether or not parents act like, and consider themselves to be, parent-partners from the get-go. The repercussions from the indifference ripple throughout society.

A legal status makes sense because if someone cannot, or will not, commit to being a parent-partner, and undertake to perform the core legal obligations that the status entails, then that person should not become a parent with the other person. Because a new automatic status would apply only to couples that had a child together *after* the new law was passed, people would know what the parent-partner status would entail and they could make an informed decision about whether and when to have a baby, and with whom.

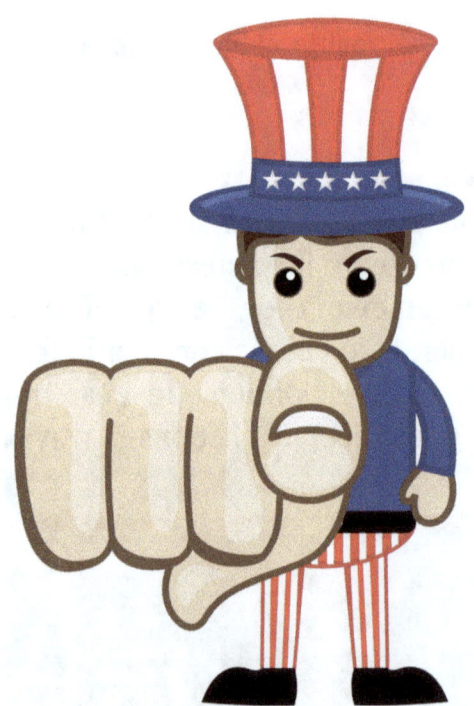

Elected representatives should create a "parent-partner" status. The status would be in addition to the existing statuses of "parent," "child," and "spouse."

The *big question* is what legal obligations should exist between parents? Perhaps you like the five obligations discussed above in the sample contract (see point 15 above)? Perhaps you have other ideas? We should be having conversations about the appropriate legal obligations. We should expect our lawmakers to be doing the same.

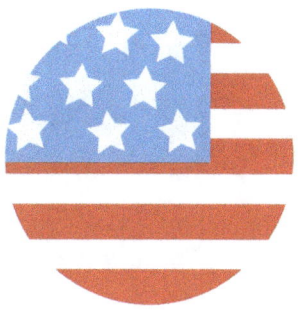

If you like the idea of a parent-partner status, you should talk to your state legislators about it. Perhaps give them a copy of this book. Family law is generally a matter of state law, and any state could create a parent-partner status.

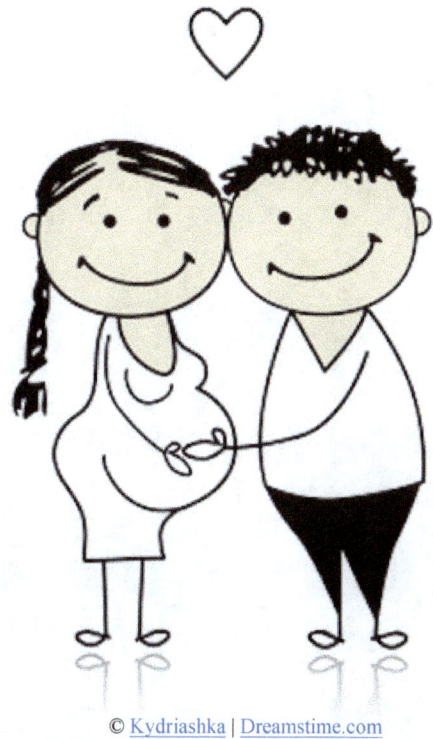

© Kydriashka | Dreamstime.com

While legal reform and social change take time, the good news is that individuals do not have to wait for the law to change before they commit to live their lives as parent-partners. Living your life as a parent-partner will advantage you, your partner, and your children. Moreover, if enough people identify as parent-partners, a social role might be created even without legal change. It is unlikely, but it is possible. So, despite the absence of a legal status for parent-partners, hopefully this book has encouraged you and your partner to live your lives as "parent-partners" and to exhibit behavior consistent with the societal expectations and legal obligations that might one day exist to accompany the new social role.

Your decision to live life as a parent-partner can have an effect on whether this idea becomes widely accepted. After all, the home can be an incubator for significant social change.

–The End–

www.ingramcontent.com/pod-product-compliance
Lightning Source LLC
Chambersburg PA
CBHW060530010526
44110CB00052B/2556